COMPLETE GUIDE TO FOAM ROLLING

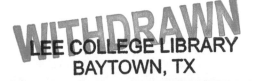

COMPLETE GUIDE TO FOAM ROLLING

Kyle Stull

DHSc, MS, LMT, CSCS, NASM-CPT, CES

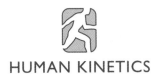

HUMAN KINETICS

Library of Congress Cataloging-in-Publication Data

Names: Stull, Kyle, 1980- author.
Title: Complete guide to foam rolling / Kyle Stull.
Description: Champaign, IL : Human Kinetics, [2018] | Includes
    bibliographical references.
Identifiers: LCCN 2017023251 (print) | LCCN 2017039591 (ebook) | ISBN
    9781492545613 (ebook) | ISBN 9781492545606 (print)
Subjects: LCSH: Exercise. | Foam rollers (Exercise equipment)
Classification: LCC RA781 (ebook) | LCC RA781 .S883 2018 (print) | DDC
    613.7/10284--DC23
LC record available at https://lccn.loc.gov/2017023251

ISBN: 978-1-4925-4560-6 (print)

Copyright © 2018 by Kyle Stull

Acquisitions Editors: Justin Klug and Michelle Maloney; **Developmental Editor:** Laura Pulliam; **Managing Editor:** Anna Lan Seaman; **Copyeditor:** Jackie Walker Gibson; **Graphic Designer:** Denise Lowry; **Cover Designer:** Keri Evans; **Photograph (cover):** Brian Fitzsimmons; **Photographs (interior):** © Human Kinetics; **Visual Production Assistant:** Joyce Brumfield; **Photo Production Manager:** Jason Allen; **Senior Art Manager:** Kelly Hendren; **Illustrations:** © Human Kinetics, unless otherwise noted; **Printer:** Versa Press

We thank TriggerPoint in Austin, Texas, for assistance in providing the location for the photo shoot for this book.

Human Kinetics books are available at special discounts for bulk purchase. Special editions or book excerpts can also be created to specification. For details, contact the Special Sales Manager at Human Kinetics.

Printed in the United States of America   10 9 8 7 6

The paper in this book is certified under a sustainable forestry program.

Human Kinetics
1607 N. Market Street
Champaign, IL 61820
USA

United States and International
Website: **US.HumanKinetics.com**
Email: info@hkusa.com
Phone: 1-800-747-4457

Canada
Website: **Canada.HumanKinetics.com**
Email: info@hkcanada.com

E6988

This book is dedicated to those who want to
improve their lives through movement. We have been given
a wonderful gift in the human body. Take care of it.

CONTENTS

Part III PROGRAMMING 125

PREFACE

This book is intended for the individual who is seeking to learn more, feel better, and move better. You may be just getting started with an exercise program, or you may be a "weekend warrior," competitive athlete, or a fitness professional hoping to gain some additional insight into foam rolling. Unfortunately, there is a lot of miscommunication about foam rolling—what it does, how to do it, why to do it, and when to do it. There is a need for consistency in the approach of applying foam rolling techniques, and foundational knowledge of the human body is mandatory.

This book will take you through this foundational knowledge and recommended techniques. You should know that this book will not make you an expert on how the body functions or teach you the molecular composition of connective tissue. However, you will be able to walk into a gym, physical therapy clinic, local running group, or your own living room and confidently apply foam rolling techniques that are safe and that will get you the best results possible. Additionally, this book will address situations when you may not need to foam roll. There are various medical conditions and injuries in which foam rolling may not be the appropriate activity or response for the body.

I decided to write this book because foam rolling has become a hot topic over the past several years. What began as a method to assist physical therapists and massage therapists more than 80 years ago (on record, anyway) has reemerged in the fitness and athletic industries as a "lifesaver," "cure-all," or "daily multivitamin" of sorts. This book will help clear up much of the confusion behind the proper use of a foam roller and provide you with programs that are based on science and approved by therapists around the world.

The concept for this book arose in my mind about 12 years ago when I first entered the fitness industry. Like many people in the fitness profession, I had my fair share of injuries. I was born with a hip condition, was routinely injured in youth sports, and in my early twenties, I was in a car accident that left me with a fractured vertebrae in my low back. Over time, all of this resulted in three reconstructive surgeries, some low back pain (not as bad as it could have been, given the situation), and chronic hip pain. While I have experienced a series of life-changing events, the first one occurred during a live workshop taught by a man named Scott Pullen with the National Academy of Sports Medicine (NASM). NASM was one of the first professional organizations not only to support the use of a foam roller, but also to teach fitness professionals how and why to use it. I had studied the material, but it wasn't until Mr.

Pullen showed me exactly how to apply the techniques that I started to notice a difference in the way I felt.

This spurring of my interest led to my pursuit of mobility and flexibility in the realm of fitness. I obtained a master of science degree with a concentration in rehabilitation and became a licensed massage therapist so I could learn more about muscles, ligaments, tendons, and fascia (connective tissue in the body). Another life-changing event occurred in 2011, when I was introduced to a company called TriggerPoint Performance (now TriggerPoint, a division of Implus LLC). TriggerPoint was founded in 2002 by Cassidy Phillips. Phillips had developed a deep tissue version of foam rolling that applied more specific techniques and had a variety of tools for different areas of the body. TriggerPoint's version of foam rolling involved a progression from the regular soft rollers. Learning this technique revealed a new world of possibilities that could be gained with a great foam roller, basic education, and specific techniques. This book will introduce many different ways to use a foam roller and discuss the pros and cons of each, hopefully leaving you with a program and roller that best fits your needs.

A series of discussions (sometimes-heated debates) with many professionals in massage therapy, physical therapy, and the fitness industry contributed greatly to this book. With each discussion, two primary concerns consistently arose: The first involved some of the terminology used with foam rolling, and the second involved the techniques people were using. Foam rolling is commonly referred to as "self-myofascial release." However, most people do not perform foam rolling even close to the way research recommends. It usually takes years to learn how to properly release muscles and connective tissue, something a highly trained professional can do. It involves identifying tight spots in muscles and applying specific techniques to change the tissue. While a foam roller may assist with this process, there is no current evidence to suggest that foam rolling releases connective tissue. So, should foam rolling be called self-myofascial release if it is not releasing the muscles and connective tissue? This book will offer a brief description of why the terms foam rolling and self-myofascial release are used interchangeably and what the future may hold.

The second concern that arose in my discussions involved how most people foam roll. People most commonly use the foam roller to select a muscle they think needs rolling and arbitrarily roll up and down for whatever time seems adequate. I have even heard a professional say, "Just roll up and down 30 to 60 times." This is wrong. A great question to ask yourself when rolling is, "What would my massage therapist do?" The answer is never to just roll up and down 30 to 60 times. They use different techniques in different directions to attempt to mobilize and change muscles. While the foam roller will never replace the thumbs of a skilled professional, it can assist and help to maintain the changes they have made.

This book is broken into three parts to help you gain a clear understanding of foam rolling and practical application of techniques. It begins with a brief overview of foam rolling, then progresses to the recommended techniques, and concludes with easy-to-follow and effective programs.

Part I will briefly explain the foundations of foam rolling. This includes the science and benefits behind rolling, some general safety recommendations, and a description of all of the equipment you will need. In addition, Part I will discuss some of the differences in the foam rolling equipment available today. With the various products that can be purchased at your local sporting goods retailer or online, it is easy to feel confused. However, all effective foam rolling tools possess a few key features.

Part II will guide you through different ways to roll each area of the body. Unfortunately, proper foam rolling is not intuitive (if it were, there would be no need for this book). While you can start anywhere, this book will suggest you begin by rolling the foot and lower leg and slowly progress up the body. Unless you have sustained a specific injury to the shoulder, there is little benefit over time to rolling only the shoulder, even if you feel shoulder pain. The body is connected from head to toe. If you move your foot while standing, the knee and hip also move. This creates motion in the spine, changes tension in the back muscles, and influences the shoulder. (Part III will help to identify the problem areas.)

Part III will begin with an explanation of how to perform a quick and easy assessment. This assessment will help you decide which areas need the most attention. While it's not a bad idea to roll the area that feels tight, it will not result in long-lasting success. It's better to learn to roll the areas that aren't moving the way they should be. Any tightness you feel may signal an area of the body that is actually moving too much and needs some stability or strengthening (not additional flexibility and stretching). Part III will also cover the different ways to foam roll based on your goals: Are you using it as a warm-up or recovery? Are you complementing a rehabilitation program from a therapist? Do you just enjoy the way it feels? While the programs may be similar, the intent makes all the difference.

This book can be read in several different ways. Of course, I suggest beginning with chapter 1 and reading all the way through. This is a great way to gain a full understanding of the concepts behind foam rolling. When using the book this way, you can understand the changes you are trying to make and roll with the intent to make those changes. However, if you want to jump to part II to get right into the techniques, you will find that each area of the body is explained in sufficient detail so that you can achieve success. You can revisit part I to learn more over time . . . or to help you fall asleep at night. Part III will provide different programs based on how you move, your goals, and your intended workout for the day (cycling, running, weightlifting programs, and so on). This section will introduce some simple movement assessments to help guide your programming. While it is not an exhaustive list, you will find several programs you can start using right away to begin to feel and move better.

Foam rolling is a tool that has helped millions of people feel better. However, you should not rely on this tool every second of every day for the rest of your life. You should also not use the foam roller as a form of treatment; if you have chronic pain or a major injury, consult a licensed health care professional. This is one of the biggest mistakes many people make. The foam roller is a tool that may feel great, and it is acceptable to use every day. However, if the only way you can make it through your run is to foam roll your leg before, during, and after the run, then you are using it to treat a symptom that has an underlying issue. This will only lead to more problems in the future.

Current research suggests that foam rolling is a great tool to use for increased range of motion and better flexibility. However, it is most effective when used with other forms of exercise. For example, foam rolling and then performing a stretch has been shown to increase range of motion better than stretching or foam rolling alone. In addition, the human body needs more than just mobility—it also needs adequate balance, stability, and coordination to function most effectively. While this book is not intended to be used for exercise, it will offer a few stretches and exercises that will add to the effectiveness of foam rolling. These will offer a great start, but if you need more information, I suggest you seek the help of a certified personal trainer.

ACKNOWLEDGMENTS

This book would not have been possible without the help of a number of people. I am thankful to be surrounded by so many who encourage growth, both personally and professionally, and who have allowed me to practice the techniques in this book on them to further refine methods of foam rolling.

First, thank you to my family for being patient as I have taken on the task of writing this book. My wife, Kandi, and daughter, Haylee, have spent many evenings and dinners with me sitting at the computer and have never complained.

Second, thank you to my many past and present work colleagues, whom I consider friends; I have learned from all of them over the years. This book is a collection of ideas and information formed only because they have given me the foundation necessary. As Isaac Newton stated, "If I have seen further, it is by standing on the shoulders of giants."

Last, but certainly not least, thank you to the hundreds of students I have had along the way who have challenged and pushed me to be better. I am amazed and humbled every day.

Part I

FOUNDATIONS

Chapter 1

SCIENCE OF FOAM ROLLING

Foam rolling is nothing new to the manual therapy world and has been used for almost 100 years in some form to support and promote health. (In fact, the first U.S. Patent filed for a handheld rolling device was in the early 1900s!) The foam roller was never and will never be intended to replace the hands of skilled therapists but rather to assist them. When used alongside therapeutic treatment, foam rolling is a great complementary tool. Massage therapists have found that when a client foam rolls between massages, their muscles feel better and they have longer-lasting results. This validates the initial theory behind foam rolling: that it could produce a similar effect to massage therapy by applying compression, encouraging circulation, and breaking up scar tissue.

As high-level athletes and Hollywood stars have begun to publicly display their foam rollers—the Denver Broncos, LeBron James, David Beckham, and Mark Wahlberg are all well-known fans of foam rolling—popularity has increased and the scientific community has shown more interest. Until recently, the question researchers have been asking is, "What does foam rolling do?" Those who use foam rollers have reported that foam rolling increases flexibility, mobility, and circulation; reduces muscle tightness and soreness; releases fascia; removes trigger points; and reduces or eliminates pain. While this type of evidence is valuable, it does not satisfy the question from a scientific perspective.

To better answer the question of the value of foam rolling, this chapter will address research that compares foam rolling to other techniques as well as the science of foam rolling before and after a workout. Additionally, this chapter will peek into some of the techniques associated with foam rolling (for example, myofascial release and trigger point therapy are often used interchangeably with foam rolling, but traditional foam rolling may not heed the same result). Lastly, this chapter will explore why foam rolling is still so misunderstood and what the future might hold.

THE RESEARCH BEHIND FOAM ROLLING

Foam rolling research is a hot topic, with a couple of studies published each month on either foam rolling or self-myofascial release. The following paragraphs take a brief look into the research on foam rolling. The intent of this information is not to overwhelm you with scientific detail but to offer an overview of findings. Application of these principles will be covered later in this book.

Foam Rolling and Flexibility

A review of literature published in *Current Sports Medicine Reports (ACSM)* (Schroeder & Best, 2015) found that foam rolling appears to have a positive effect on flexibility before exercise and results in decreased soreness and fatigue following exercise. Many studies compare foam rolling to another tool or stretching technique. For example, researchers Skarabot, Beardsley, and Stirn (2015) compared foam rolling to traditional stretching, and the results suggested that both stretching and foam rolling can increase flexibility. However, to gain the most flexibility, participants needed to use a combination of both foam rolling and stretching. Participants who foam rolled for one minute before stretching had the best results.

Similarly, researcher Goran Markovic (2015) compared foam rolling to a therapist's use of a handheld tool on hip and knee motion in soccer players. Markovic found that both foam rolling and the handheld tool improve the motion at the hip and knee. It should be noted that the foam rolling group was able to perform the rolling by themselves and the other group had to have a therapist apply the tool. This is significant because foam rolling is a self-application technique. The true value is that people can do it themselves and not rely on others to help.

Foam Rolling and Performance

Foam rolling has been found to be an effective tool before a workout. According to a review of literature published in *Current Sports Medicine Reports (ACSM)* (Schroeder & Best, 2015), foam rolling appears to have a positive effect on flexibility before exercise and decreases soreness and fatigue following exercise. These findings suggest that foam rolling affects performance.

Similarly, researcher Cheatham and colleagues (2015) concluded that foam rolling is effective at increasing the ability of joints to move and improving performance. In another study by Peacock and colleagues (2014), foam rolling before basic performance testing (such as jumping, agility drills, and heavy weightlifting) increased performance. The best results were found among participants who foam rolled followed by stretching that mimicked the workout (also referred to as dynamic stretching).

Lanigan and Harrison (2012) found that foam rolling the bottom of the foot may increase jump height. Several studies have supported this notion. Even when foam rolling has not been shown to increase jump height, it also did not decrease jump height. While researchers have not yet demonstrated why foam rolling can sometimes increase jump height, the finding can likely be attributed to the positive effect of foam rolling on overall movement: If one area of the body can move optimally, then surrounding muscles may fire better. When one muscle contracts, the muscle on the opposite side of the joint relaxes.

In a nervous system that's functioning optimally, this mechanism works great and allows us to efficiently move from point A to point B. However, if a muscle is stuck in a shortened position, which is frequently the case, then the muscle on the opposite side of the joint cannot contract when needed. Consider walking, running, or performing any number of activities that require the hips to move. During optimal function, someone can use their glutes to propel forward. However, if someone has a shortened hip flexor (the muscle opposite the glutes), then the glutes cannot fully contract. They are inhibited. Performance is likely to decrease, and the chance of injury is likely to increase. If this same person used a foam roller to decrease tension and tightness in the hip flexor, it would increase the ability of the glutes to contract, thereby increasing performance and decreasing the chance of a hamstring injury.

Foam rolling has also been shown to reduce fatigue when performed before a workout (Healey et al., 2013). A reduction in fatigue could lead to more enjoyment during training, more consistency, and better results overall.

One consistent theme that emerges from the current research is that foam rolling before exercise does not appear to negatively affect performance. To further support these findings, reputable organizations such as the National Academy of Sports Medicine, TriggerPoint, and Functional Movement Systems have encouraged the use of a foam roller before exercise for more than a decade.

Foam rolling has also proven to serve as a great cool-down after a workout. Researchers MacDonald and colleagues (2014) found that foam rolling after heavy weightlifting can speed up recovery, decrease soreness, and help improve performance on many tests (such as jump height). The participants performed heavy squats and then foam rolled. They returned to the research lab 24 hours later to measure soreness and repeat performance testing. In the days following the heavy squats, the foam rolling group's soreness peaked at 24 hours, whereas the non-foam rolling group's soreness peaked at 48 hours. Pearcy and colleagues (2015) supported the finding that foam rolling after intense exercise can decrease the soreness that occurs 24- to 48-hours after a workout, while also increasing performance. It is important to note that many participants did experience soreness in both of these studies, but the soreness was not as severe and appeared to dissipate more quickly when compared to those who did not foam roll. This suggests that soreness after an intense workout is likely, but foam rolling may improve the body's ability to recover. Edmunds and colleagues (2016) performed a study to explore the difference in muscle recovery after a workout. One group of participants foam rolled and another performed traditional stretching. The researchers found that foam rolling may help maintain muscle force the following day when compared to stretching. Collectively this research on foam rolling after exercise suggests that spending just a few minutes foam rolling after a workout can have a huge impact on how quickly someone recovers.

Foam Rolling and the Heart

Research on foam rolling also goes beyond performance and flexibility. Okamoto, Masuhara, and Ikuta (2014) found that foam rolling also helped the heart. Participants in the study used a foam roller on various body parts for one minute each. The result was an increase in the flexibility of the arteries in the muscle groups that were rolled. The arteries are responsible for carrying oxygen-rich blood from the heart throughout the body. Arteries have thick, elastic, and muscular walls that can become stiff, similar to other muscles. Therefore, the more flexible the artery is, the better it can help push blood through the body. While the research did not test veins, which have a different structure (thin, non-elastic), foam rolling may also be beneficial to veins because the pressure can increase circulation. Once blood has delivered its oxygen to the muscle, the veins carry it back to the heart and lungs. Veins contain small valves that prevent the back flow or pooling of blood in one particular area. Varicose veins occur when the valve does not properly function and the blood pools to one area, causing weakening and expansion of the vein. Foam rolling varicose veins is not advised and will be discussed in a chapter 3. However, foam rolling may help to prevent some varicose veins if used regularly.

Foam Rolling and the Nervous System

The last foam rolling effect to consider is the potential for other physiological changes. Up to this point, the discussion of research has been around physical changes such as performance, recovery, soreness, and fatigue. However, in one of the first textbooks to speak on foam rolling, *Integrated Training for the New Millennium* (2000), Dr. Michael Clark suggested that foam rolling may also be a tool that works on the nervous system. Dr. Clark further elaborated on this concept in 2011, writing that using a foam roller to place slow or sustained pressure onto a muscle can stimulate certain receptors that communicate with the nervous system, causing the muscle to relax. The research on nervous system effects stems from changes noticed on clients during massage. Chan and colleagues (2015) studied how self-massage may affect the nervous system. The participants in this study experienced chronic pain. They were taught how to perform self-massage to the painful area and given home exercises to perform. The self-massage program involved using a hard ball and holding pressure on uncomfortable spots. Researchers found that patients who performed self-massage increased the relaxation side of the nervous system, thereby reducing overall stress. This study supported older research in which a therapist held pressure on painful spots (Delaney et al., 2002; Takamoto et al., 2009). These two studies were performed by massage therapists but had a similar effect of reducing fatigue and stress.

While massage therapy and foam rolling have similarities, there are also significant differences. For example, therapists are highly skilled at finding tight spots in muscles and helping to relax their clients. Foam rolling requires self-inflicted discomfort. Thus, the results may be highly variable. In 2014, Kim and colleagues suggested that self-myofascial release did not lead to the reduction of stress. A primary difference between this study and the others is that these participants were considered healthy and performed a light 30-minute workout before foam rolling. The previous studies included participants that dealt with chronic pain.

Foam Rolling and Myofascial Release

Foam rolling is often referred to as self-myofascial release—in other words, myofascial release that people do for themselves. Therefore, the question often arises, "What is myofascial release, and is foam rolling the same thing?"

Myofascia is a combination of two words: "myo" means muscle, and "fascia" is defined as connective tissue in the body. Connective tissues are tissues like tendons and ligaments that simply serve to connect muscles and do not work to produce force and movement. Fascia is a connective tissue that expands throughout the body. It can surround organs and muscles, appear in between muscles, and even connect to the skin. This fascia serves the purpose of supporting many different movements and positions. For example, someone who has performed heavy lifting for many years is likely to have thickened fascia in the areas of the body that do the most work. This thickening is an effort to make the body more efficient at the heavy lifting. Likewise, a marathon runner is likely to have thickening in the fascia around the calves and thighs. Every time the foot hits the ground, the muscles contract to help propel the body forward. This increases stress to the connective tissue (fascia), and over time it becomes thicker to make running more efficient. Conversely, if someone spends more time sitting—not using their body and not applying stress to the fascia—it may become thin, weak, and prone to injury.

An important thing to remember is that muscle and fascia always work together. The muscle contracts and the fascia supports, ultimately to produce desired movement. A variety of factors can damage muscle and fascia (myofascia). Some of the most common are dehydration and overuse or repetitive movement. When damaged or stressed too much, the myofascia may respond by laying down extra tissue, similar to a scar. If too much scar tissue forms, it begins to restrict movement and may cause pain either in the direct area or surrounding areas.

Myofascial release is a hands-on technique performed by licensed and usually highly skilled manual therapists such as a doctor of physical therapy, a doctor of chiropractic, or a licensed massage therapist. It has been defined by myofascial therapist Mark Barnes (1997) as a method of finding restricted (damaged) tissue and holding pressure onto the area until a release is felt, which often occurs around 90 seconds. After the first release, the therapist continues to hold pressure, albeit slightly more, until a second release is felt. This process may be repeated for up to several minutes. Theories suggest that the changes occur because the fascia can become better hydrated. This causes the fascia to soften, becoming more of a gel as compared to a solid. The scar tissue, while never completely eliminated, realigns to support movement better. Myofascial release has been highly regarded as a practical and effective method of reducing pain and restoring function for many individuals. The question remains, can foam rolling reproduce this effect to restore the fascia?

There is no current evidence either supporting or denying the role of foam rolling in myofascial release. However, many myofascial therapists suggest that a partial replication is possible. This would be performed by slowly rolling a foam roller across a muscle, searching for a tender spot (which would represent restricted or damaged tissue). Then, pressure would be sustained on that spot until a release or a reduction in tenderness is felt. This would represent the "first barrier releasing," as suggested by Mark Barnes (1997). Next, pressure would be sustained in the same spot to address the next barrier, and the process may repeat for several minutes. Two primary concerns arise when using a foam roller for myofascial release: (1) Myofascial therapists are experts at finding restricted tissue, whereas the average person using a foam roller may not know what this feels like. (2) Few people want to lie on a foam roller for several minutes. So, to answer the question, foam rolling has the potential to work similarly to myofascial release, but often foam rolling does not create myofascial release due to improper use.

Foam Rolling and Trigger Points

Foam rolling began as a tool to reduce the negative side effects associated with trigger points. The National Academy of Sports Medicine, which introduced foam rolling to the health and fitness industry in 2000, referred to this impact on trigger points as self-myofascial release. That notion was later supported in 2002 by TriggerPoint founder Cassidy Phillips. Trigger points, sometimes called myofascial trigger points, are irritable spots in muscles that are painful when pressed (Travell, Simons, & Simons, 1999). People typically experience these irritable spots in similar muscles, and the irritable spots often have a distinct pain pattern. For example, when a trigger point in the neck or shoulder muscles is pressed, the person may feel pain through the neck and around the head. This is a common trapezius trigger point. The problem with trigger points is not only that they hurt, but also that they cause the muscles to be in a continuous state of fatigue. A muscle that has trigger points is usually chronically contracted for some reason. It may be that the muscle has been stuck in a shortened position after the person has been in a cast. Or the muscles may have been chronically lengthened in an attempt to support a part of the body. Essentially, the body decides that it is better for a particular muscle to be chronically tense, so it places a hyperirritable bundle of tissue there to support the position.

Trigger point release is usually performed by a licensed massage therapist who is specifically trained to work with trigger points. A common method is to apply pressure directly on or near the trigger point to disrupt blood and oxygen flow. When this decreases, the trigger point may weaken or relax, allowing the muscle to be stretched and further decreasing the trigger point. The foam roller can be used in much the same way. A person can apply pressure directly to a tender spot. By holding pressure, it will decrease the blood and

UNDERSTANDING THE MISUNDERSTANDING ABOUT FOAM ROLLING

With all the information available on foam rolling, why is it still done improperly and why do people rarely realize the full benefit? There is not a clear answer to this, but let's consider intuition. Foam rollers are cylinders, and cylinders roll. Therefore, it makes sense to get on the ground and roll. However, rolling is usually painful or uncomfortable. Who would want to roll slowly and spend up to several minutes doing something that hurts? What ends up happening is that people get on the foam roller, roll as quickly as possible, and stop before any real changes occur. To be fair, the science behind foam rolling suggests that any rolling is better than no rolling for most people. So, a person who spends 20 seconds rolling an entire upper leg will feel better than before they started. Researchers Sullivan and colleagues (2013) had participants roll the hamstrings incredibly fast. The entire length of the muscle was rolled at a pace of 120 beats per minute. At this speed the roller was traveling from the hips to the knee and back in one second. Different groups performed the rolling at the same speed but different lengths of time. No group performed the rolling for longer than 20 seconds total. The groups increased flexibility in the muscle, but (and this is a big but) the changes lasted less than 10 minutes!

The moral of the story is that to maximize the benefit and value of foam rolling, it's important to follow the suggested programming from the experts. Spend time on the areas of the body that need it. Foam roll before and after a workout, breathe as you roll, and allow the muscle to relax. While you're likely to feel better quickly, this is not something that is intended to be an immediate change. You didn't get tight overnight.

oxygen supply. After a period of time (the time may vary per individual), the trigger point will relax allowing the muscle to be stretched, further reducing the trigger point. An important note here is that many trigger points lie in the deep muscles that are difficult for the average foam roller to reach. In these cases, it is great to have a therapist and a variety of foam rolling products to try to get deeper. Additionally, the constant back-and-forth rolling that so many have become accustomed to will not reduce or eliminate trigger points. It is imperative that the user stop on the tender spots, hold, and breathe until there is some sort of reduction in pain or tenderness.

While foam rolling may help reduce the negative side effects of trigger points or possibly prevent trigger points, it will not eliminate trigger points on its own. Trigger points form due to some form of trauma or prolonged stress. This could be the result of an injury, or it may just be from months or years of improper posture. Take, for example, the office worker who has spent a significant amount of time sitting at a desk slouched over a keyboard. The stress placed on the muscles of the upper back and shoulders becomes too much for the body. It is common for trigger points to form in these areas. Using a foam roller on the upper back may feel great, but it will do little to reduce the trigger points until posture is fixed. The bottom line is that foam rolling is a great tool, but it may not fix everything. A quick assessment will be performed in chapter 10, but if you have questions regarding this, it is always advisable and helpful to speak to a health and fitness professional.

THE FUTURE OF FOAM ROLLING RESEARCH

Foam rolling research has come a long way in recent years. However, the future has a lot in store. While the majority of research has suggested that it is beneficial for movement by increasing flexibility, range of motion, and some performance; helps reduce pain from higher intensity workouts; and speeds recovery, no research study has really proven what foam rolling actually does. Many of the research articles cited in this book have conclusions with theories on why it works. For example, in the Sullivan and colleagues (2013) study with the really fast rolling (120 beats per minute), the authors concluded by suggesting that the high rates of rolling could have induced so much friction and heat that it broke up scar tissue and small adhesions that had formed between muscles. Maybe this is why the participants had better flexibility. Other articles suggest that the increased blood flow may have to do with the improvements in flexibility and performance or that the mere enjoyment of or distaste for foam rolling may be the reason for the changes. For example, Healey and colleagues (2013) state that foam rolling before exercise may reduce fatigue during a workout and that "the subjects' perception of how they liked or disliked using the foam roller could have altered how well they performed . . . ." Perhaps someone loves foam rolling, and this gets them excited about their workout. Conversely, someone hates foam rolling, and this excites him or her, allowing the person to workout harder and longer. No studies have looked into this in detail. It is simply an interesting consideration.

At the time of this writing, foam roller manufacturer TriggerPoint is conducting research with universities to find out more about why foam rolling actually works. In an unpublished pilot study at the University of Texas in 2013, researchers Fleisher and colleagues found that using a foam roller on the calf muscle resulted in increased blood flow up the thigh. This is interesting because it was the first look at circulation in an area away from where the foam rolling occurred. While more research needs to be conducted, this could provide insight into the circulation question, suggesting that foam rolling does indeed increase blood flow through the body.

Additional studies are looking into pain pressure threshold (does foam rolling increase the amount of pain one can tolerate, thus allowing them to do more?); localized flood blow (how much blood flow increase occurs at the muscles being rolled?); myofascial release (can foam rolling actually release connective tissue?); other uses for foam rolling (can foam rolling be an effective method to help treat medical conditions such as plantar fasciitis or low-back pain?); and balance (does foam rolling help improve balance in the elderly?). In the next two years, it is likely that these questions, along with many others, will be answered.

Foam rolling has taken the health, wellness, and sports industries by storm over the past several years. Professional athletes and everyday athletes are getting in on the fun by investing in different types of rollers and seeking out more information. While some of the scientific research does not fully support the use of a foam roller, most do. No one knows exactly why yet, but it appears that rolling is better than not rolling. Scientific research is continuing to emerge around this topic and will soon suggest more specific types of rollers and specific ways to use them. Now that the current scientific research has been introduced, the next chapter will discuss what all of this means in terms of the benefits.

Chapter 2

BENEFITS OF FOAM ROLLING

The previous chapter took a look at the current science and research surrounding foam rolling. The more research is performed around foam rolling, the more prestige and attention the practice will receive in the scientific and medical communities. However, many of the benefits of foam rolling are things that can't be quantified. Thus, they are not easily measured in a lab and may never end up in a scientific journal. This chapter will explain the benefits of foam rolling, based on the research mentioned in the previous chapter. The chapter will conclude by discussing a few case studies that have been presented but will likely never make it to a lab or a journal: for example, use of the foam roller to reduce pain and stay active, foam rolling effects that can last up to 36 hours, and the foam roller's temporary reduction of blood pressure.

BENEFITS OF FOAM ROLLING BEFORE, DURING, AND AFTER A WORKOUT

Foam rolling adds value to many different exercise regimens and daily activities. It does not have to take up a considerable portion of your day or even much of your workout. In most cases, rolling just a few muscles for a few minutes is adequate to achieve the benefits. If foam rolling in a health club, you can take their roller and a mat to a corner. This is actually a great way to relax and get ready if you're about to work out or to relax after a workout. If you're at home preparing for a run, you can spend a few minutes foam rolling while finishing up your favorite show. Let's take a closer look at these workout benefits.

Before a Workout

Foam rolling just makes sense as part of a cool-down. However, foam rolling is also incredibly valuable when performed before a workout. Chapter 1 highlighted several research studies that found that foam rolling increases flexibility (how well muscles can stretch and shorten). The better flexibility a muscle has, the better movement will be at the joints. Not everyone needs more flexibility, and having too much flexibility could set you up for injuries. However, most adults could stand to increase flexibility in at least some muscles. A common reason for injuries during a workout is stiffness or tightness. If a muscle can't fully extend, yet is forced to, there is a potential for it to become injured or slightly damaged, thus leading to soreness. For example, consider taking up running after years of sitting at a desk. To run properly the hip needs to be able to fully extend as the foot is pushing off the ground, thus demonstrating flexibility.

However, after years of sitting, the muscles in the front of the hips become short and stuck. It's unlikely they will be able to fully lengthen and pull the low back into an extended position, known as lumbar hyperextension (see figure 2.1). It is common for the runner with tight hips to not feel it in the hips but to end up having some low-back pain or maybe even knee soreness after beginning a running program. They will likely chalk it up to "being out of shape," or they may say, "running is bad for their joints." In reality, their hips are restricting proper motion, disrupting the body's natural ability to absorb force and resulting in aches and pains in a different part of the body. Spending a few minutes foam rolling before a workout can increase flexibility to these tight spots, allowing them to extend properly, increasing flexibility, and prepping them for the workout to come.

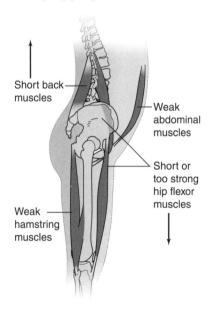

Short back muscles

Weak abdominal muscles

Short or too strong hip flexor muscles

Weak hamstring muscles

Figure 2.1 Lumbar hyperextension.

Foam rolling can also increase circulation. One of the main purposes of a warm-up is to get the blood flowing and the fluids moving. Areas commonly injured during a workout—such as tendons, ligaments, and other connective tissues—may not receive adequate blood flow. Areas that usually enjoy a lot of blood flow aren't injured as frequently. Foam rolling can increase total body circulation, but it has a greater circulation effect locally. On days when your workout involves a lot of lower body exercises, foam rolling the legs (calves, hamstrings, quads, and glutes) can help move blood and fluid to all the tissues. This reduces the chance of minor sprains and strains during a normal workout.

Additionally, chapter 1 noted that foam rolling could help increase mobility. Mobility often goes hand-in-hand with flexibility—but they are different. Flexibility is usually specific to extensibility of muscles and mobility is commonly used to describe how joints move. Flexibility may affect mobility, and mobility may affect flexibility. For example, if the quadriceps in the fronts of the legs are tight, the knee will show less mobility. Likewise, if the knee has arthritis and does not demonstrate ideal mobility, over time the quadriceps will become tight and lose flexibility. Because foam rolling increases flexibility of the muscles, your mobility can also increase.

The body is designed to move in many different directions with many muscles contributing. If joints or muscles can't move—and therefore have limited mobility and flexibility—then the muscles can't generate the force they are capable of and performance is likely to decrease. Consider the jump squat, as shown in figure 2.2. In order for the muscles to generate the maximum amount of force, they must be able to lengthen and shorten fully. If one

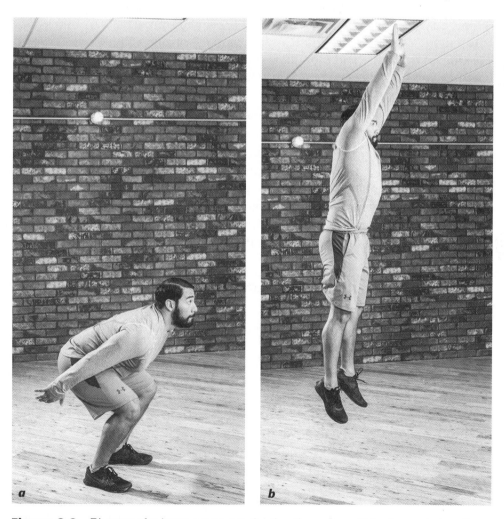

Figure 2.2 Phases of a jump squat emphasize the value of ideal muscle length.

Note: In order to get to the bottom position correctly, the muscles of the lower leg and upper leg must lengthen (a). Additionally, to get maximum height, the muscles of the shoulders must lengthen (b).

muscle is short and tight, then somewhere else in the body there is a muscle that is long. Whether shortened or lengthened, muscles that are out of optimal alignment are weaker.

Keeping the muscles and joints moving may help increase performance, but as noted in chapter 1, while research suggests foam rolling may not always increase performance, there has never been a decrease in performance shown. As will be discussed in chapter 11, the best way to integrate foam rolling into a workout is to perform it before a dynamic warm-up routine. In this scenario, the foam rolling helps the body move better, and then some bodyweight exercises prepare the body to perform at its peak.

Chapter 1 also noted that foam rolling before a workout may decrease fatigue. During a workout the body is expending a great deal of energy; after a period of time, everyone begins to get a little tired. Research has not yet concluded exactly why foam rolling may reduce fatigue, but it is likely that foam rolling helps properly prepare the body for a workout. The warm-up is not only a time to get the body physically prepared—by increasing blood flow and working on flexibility and mobility—but also a time to get mentally prepared. Foam rolling correctly can help you relax, focus on your body, and breathe in lots of fresh oxygen. These few minutes spent breathing and concentrating on how each muscle feels can go a long way in a workout.

During a Workout

While not discussed in chapter 1, rolling during a workout is also a great use of foam rolling. One of the biggest mistakes people make in an exercise program is how they address the rest period, or the amount of time they take between exercises. In order for exercise to have an effect on the body, the rest period should be based on the intensity of the workout. If you are lifting as much weight as possible or sprinting as fast as possible, you will need to rest for at least a couple of minutes to let your energy restore before repeating the exercise. If energy is not properly restored, the level of intensity must be reduced. If you are working out with a very low intensity, lifting a low amount of weight, or doing slow cardio, you may not need any rest.

So the question becomes this: If you do indeed need a rest period, what should you do? "Rest" means something different for everyone, but during a workout, it means anything that is at a lower intensity than the exercise. It doesn't mean sit around and talk—in fact, many health and fitness professionals don't allow their clients to sit at all. Instead, the time should be used to allow the heart rate to come back down a few beats per minute, allow the oxygen to flow through the muscles, and allow our main energy source to begin to replenish. This can be achieved with a light jog, a brisk walk, some moderate stretching, or foam rolling. It would be more appropriate to call this period "active recovery," instead of pure "rest."

Integrating foam rolling into a workout is especially great if you are performing exercises as a circuit, or "circuit training." Circuit training involves performing several exercises sequentially in a series. This may mean alternating upper and lower body exercises or possibly working the same body part through different exercises. Circuit training almost always allows some time for rest or recovery. A common and very effective method of using foam rolling as part of an active recovery is to use the roller on muscles that tend to become "tight" or short during a workout. For example, it is common for people to have short muscles in their calves. Certain shoes or even the way someone walks can affect these muscles. If you want to perform lower-body exercises but your calves always feel "tight" after squats, lunges, or jumps, you can prevent or offset the tightness by foam rolling. Simply foam roll and stretch the calves as part of the warm-up; then after each set, roll the calves for about 30 seconds as the heart rate decreases and the muscles refuel. (This may actually help the other muscles to work better too.)

Another common issue occurs when people want to tone the glutes—this is especially true when summer is approaching. The glutes are an important muscle to address in some cases of low back pain. However, again due to lifestyle, the hips are often so tight that people can't get their glutes to work properly. If your hips are tight, you could foam roll and stretch the problematic muscles of the hips before the workout. You could also plan to foam roll during the workout, thereby maximizing the amount of work the other muscles are able to do.

Remember the discussion about how when one muscle tightens, it affects the other muscles? This is the perfect example. After performing exercises that work a target area, spend 30 to 60 seconds rolling and maybe even stretching the muscles on the other side of the joint. Take the deadlift, which is an excellent strength exercise for the glutes and hamstrings. If the muscle on the front of the hip (hip flexor) is short and tight, it will decrease the ability of the glutes to contract. So, after a set of deadlifts, instead of resting in a seated position that shortens the hip flexor, grab your foam roller and spend 30 seconds rolling and stretching out each side. The same is true for the upper body. If you want a better back, spend some time foam rolling and stretching your front.

After a Workout

Foam rolling can have benefits after a workout as well. Chapter 1 introduced research about the ability of the foam roller to reduce soreness if used as part of a cool-down. Fitness enthusiasts may want to reduce soreness quickly so that they can complete a harder workout more frequently. Others may want to reduce soreness so they simply won't be as uncomfortable for as long after exercise.

Soreness after exercise comes from microscopic tears in the muscles. This is a natural part of the adaptation process where the muscles experience damage, and our amazing body comes back and repairs them to be stronger and bigger than they were before. One of the most important aspects of this repair is proper recovery. The muscles need nutrients that are provided through the blood. The quicker the nutrients are brought to the muscle, the quicker the body can recover. A few minutes spent foam rolling the muscles that did the most work (thus, the ones more likely to need more nutrients), the quicker that recovery process will begin and the quicker the damage will be fixed. It should be noted, however, that soreness is not all bad—it is simply a sign that the muscles did more than they have in a long time.

Regularly foam rolling after a workout may have a longer effect than just reducing soreness. When the muscles experience microscopic damage, they repair themselves by lying down additional tissue and regrowing stronger. This process is similar to how a scar forms after a cut. After too many days, weeks, months, or even years without proper stretching and muscle maintenance, the muscles may begin to shorten or the tissue may harden and become resistant to normal movement. For example, after a surgery, many therapists believe that scar tissue can be easily stretched until about 12 weeks, at which point it may become too hard and thick to demonstrate normal movement. The shortening and hardening is a simple response to the regrowth when the body is not achieving proper flexibility and mobility. The short muscles may not only feel uncomfortable, but they could also increase the potential for injury. Muscles are supposed to maintain an ideal length where they can provide the best support for posture and movement. However, when muscles on one side of a joint begin to shorten, the muscles on the other side of the joint are forced to lengthen. This less-than-ideal relationship between the muscles can add additional stress to the joint, which increases the chance of repetitive strain injuries. Foam rolling after a workout, as part of the cool-down routine, may prevent much of this tightness and muscle imbalance. In order to get the most amount of muscle length, Skarabot, Beardsley, and Stirn (2015) found foam rolling followed by static stretching yielded the best results.

PHYSIOLOGICAL BENEFITS OF FOAM ROLLING

Foam rolling can affect many different systems within the body. If used correctly, it can play a role in the nervous system, decreasing tension and stress, and may even help with pain. Let's take a look at some of the physiological benefits.

Foam Rolling and Its Effect on the Central Nervous System

Foam rolling can also positively affect the nervous system. As was mentioned in chapter 1, the pressure on receptors in the body may induce relaxation. These receptors are located throughout the body and are closely connected to the nervous system. They communicate information about tension or stress on the muscles, and in some cases they signal pain. Anyone who has ever had a massage has likely experienced this relaxation. By applying and holding pressure for a period of time (the time varies per individual), it is possible to generate a relaxation effect. That effect results in better blood flow, decreased heart rate, decreased blood pressure, better breathing, and reduced overall stress. Dr. Clark, former CEO of the National Academy of Sports Medicine, suggested that foam rolling be used for two primary reasons, and one of these reasons is to reduce tension in the body (Clark & Lucett, 2011). While the research was based on findings from manual therapy, such as massage, foam rolling may have the same effect if done correctly. If we consider the proper use of foam rolling, applying pressure slowly into a muscle as you concentrate on your breathing seems to almost always have a relaxing effect, even if research has yet to prove it. Additionally, this decrease in tension and stress may explain why some people feel less fatigue and experience more enjoyment of the workout after foam rolling.

Foam Rolling and Its Effect on Myofascial Release

As discussed in chapter 1, myofascial release involves release of the muscle and fascia, or connective tissue. Let's explore the benefits of releasing the myofascial (which go hand-in-hand with the flexibility and mobility benefits discussed previously). When the fascia system moves better, the body feels and moves better. However, the health of fascia should be thought of differently than the health of muscle because fascia and muscle are different. For example, a muscle can contract in an instant, whereas fascia cannot. Fascia responds to longer and slower pressure on the body and certain chemicals, such as stress hormones. If you are lifting heavy boxes every day for several months, then the fascia in the low back will slowly contract as stress is placed on the muscles. Essentially, the fascia is contracting to help you continue lifting heavy boxes; it is reinforcing a habit—whether good or bad. Reinforcing the habit of lifting heavy boxes is great when you're lifting heavy boxes, but it will not feel great if you decide to go golfing and need that fascia in the low back to move well. Just as fascia will slowly contract over time if stressed, releasing the fascia is also a slow process and must be done along with movement.

Fascia is, in large part, water. Pressure from the foam roller will "squeeze" water out of the cells in the fascia. Then when the pressure is removed, the water will be "sucked" back up into the cells. This slow but steady process can infuse more water into the cells than was previously there. Why is this important? When the fascia is dehydrated, it is sticky, like mucus. Thus, instead of moving and sliding freely, it sticks. When stuck, it generates more friction, which initiates a downward cycle of dysfunction. But when fascia is hydrated, it is smooth and frictionless, allowing the body to generate force and stabilize.

Foam Rolling and Its Effect on Trigger Point Release

As explained in chapter 1, trigger points are hyperirritable muscle fibers. They develop for a variety of reasons, but what they have in common is that most of them hurt—especially when the muscle in which the trigger point resides contracts to shorten or stretches out. Additionally, as discussed in chapter 1, trigger points can often refer pain to other places in the body. These other areas aren't random as they follow a particular pattern, which previous research has identified.

To most people trigger points feel like little "knots" or bumps in the muscle. Getting rid of them can often provide great relief. The tricky thing about trigger points is that the body may have them for a very specific reason. Releasing them may not always be the best thing to do. One area that commonly experiences tightness and pain related to trigger points is the upper shoulders and neck, a result of the very common forward head position discussed in chapter 1. This area may not only require some foam rolling, but also require an exercise routine that strengthens the appropriate muscles and reinforces proper posture. Only then will the trigger points actually go away.

After a trigger point is released or eliminated then the muscles can more easily and freely lengthen and shorten, without feeling painful. It is very common for a muscle that has trigger points to also be short. Therefore, after doing some foam rolling, some stretching may be necessary to completely eliminate the trigger point. If you believe you have trigger points, it is recommended to speak to a professional who is trained in trigger point therapy. Chapter 3 also covers areas of the body where caution should be used.

Foam Rolling and Its Effect on Pain

When it comes to pain, the benefits of foam rolling can be difficult to quantify. Some of the more recent research around pain, especially chronic pain, is focused on the context of pain (Butler & Moseley, 2013). Your environment can play a huge role in the effects of an injury. Imagine someone who has been shot in the leg in war. This is a stressful situation in which adrenaline and other hormones are coursing through the body. You may have heard stories where the person does not even realize she has been shot. On the other hand, a simple paper cut can have you in tears! How can these two injuries feel so different? The answer lies in the context in which they occurred.

Theories surrounding the effects of foam rolling on pain consider this idea. While use of the foam roller on an area that has persistent pain may not always release tissue or eliminate all of the trigger points, it will change the information that is being relayed to the brain (in other words, information about the context in which the pain is being felt). To think of this a little differently, consider your response if you were to bump your elbow while walking through a doorway. What would be one of your first responses? Some may have a couple of choice words to say, but it's likely you would rub your elbow. Your intuition is to rub the elbow to change the context of the moment: The rubbing introduces movement where there was once pain, and the brain has to decide which is more important at the time. To apply this theory to foam rolling, consider the example of an avid runner who is experiencing chronic pain from a tight iliotibial band (the thick band of fascia that runs from the hip to the shin along the outside of the knee); foam rolling it, even for a few seconds, is likely to eliminate or greatly reduce the pain because it changes the context of the pain. This is a brilliant use of foam rolling as long as the user understands that he or she is merely buying a little extra time and is not addressing the root cause. Pain in the iliotibial band is usually the result of an imbalance in the hips. Therefore, while rolling the iliotibial band may provide some relief, other areas must also be rolled and the root cause must be addressed.

HOW LONG DO THE BENEFITS OF FOAM ROLLING LAST?

While there are many benefits of foam rolling, the research on how long these benefits will last is unclear because there has been such a variety in how each participant foam rolls. Recall from chapter 1 that rolling incredibly quickly results in increased flexibility without a decrease in performance— but the changes only last 10 minutes. However, a couple of surveys I have conducted along with TriggerPoint have suggested something much different. A group of professional cyclists in Tuscon, Arizona, during spring training camps, foam rolled on their non-dominant legs 24 hours before a semi-long training ride. They rolled the calves, quadriceps, glutes, and psoas major (toward the base of the vertebrae and top of the pelvis); they did not roll or stretch their dominant legs in any way before the ride. Upon completion of the ride, they took a small survey to describe how their legs felt. Almost all of the participants said the leg that was rolled "felt stronger" and had "less fatigue" compared to their otherwise stronger leg. In another survey, a group of 20 amateur hikers near Santa Monica, California, worked with a certified personal trainer to foam roll the same areas as the cyclists. The hikers also rolled the upper back and chest muscles on the non-dominant side of the body. Here, the foam rolling occurred 36 hours before the hike began. Upon conclusion of the hike, participants answered questions about how they felt, and their answers were the same as the cyclists: The hikers said that the leg that had been foam rolled "felt better" than the leg that was not foam rolled. While this is very anecdotal and only included a small number of participants overall, it is great pilot data to encourage researchers to take a better and more detailed look at how long these effects last. It should be noted that the participants could not necessarily explain why things felt better. There was nothing specific that stood out between the two legs during physical activity other than just feeling a little better, a little stronger, and less fatigued after the activity.

Finding the Benefits in Frequency and Consistency

It is rare that someone stands up after foam rolling and says, "I love foam rolling so much!" It is more common to hear someone say, "Why would I do that again?" because foam rolling can sometimes be uncomfortable. However, the pain and discomfort is not necessarily the goal of foam rolling. (If the pain is extreme, you can switch to a softer roller or change your position.) Rather, you can achieve the benefits discussed in this chapter by creating consistency in your rolling routine. The body adapts to exercise over time. The only way this occurs is if the stimulus (such as weightlifting, cardio, or stretching) is consistently performed. Foam rolling is similar. While the benefits of foam rolling are often immediately realized, in order for the muscles and other tissues to change permanently, you must foam roll regularly.

Consider what it is your body does every day: Are you using it to its full capacity, allowing it to recover properly, keeping it hydrated, and feeding it all the nutrients it needs to rebuild and repair? Few people in today's society are doing this. If you are not giving your body what it needs daily, you may need to perform foam rolling more frequently and for longer periods each time. TriggerPoint founder Cassidy Phillips has compared foam rolling to brushing teeth. Phillips has often been heard saying, "You brush your teeth every day to keep the plaque from building up, and you need to 'brush' your muscles every day to keep the gunk from building up." While muscles do not accumulate plaque the same as teeth, the analogy rings true. Foam rolling consistently will help keep the tissues hydrated, moving smoothly across each other, and prevent them from getting stuck, short, and tight.

So far no one has performed a study to determine how frequently foam rolling should be performed. However, many experts in the field have suggested that three times per week would be a minimum for maintenance and once a day would be ideal if there is a specific problem that needs to be addressed. The best thing to do is to consider your lifestyle: What kinds of shoes do you wear? How much do you sit every day? How hard do you work out? All of these factors play a role in the degree of wear and tear the body experiences. It is quite possible you may need to roll twice a day to help initiate the change and then once per day to maintain it.

Take knee pain, for example. Imagine your doctor has concluded you do not have any torn muscles or ligaments in the knee and suggests you lightly stretch the calves. If you have an office job where you work eight hours per day, you may be required to wear business casual clothes, including a shoe with an elevated heel. An elevated heel shortens the calf muscles. If you wear those shoes for extended periods of time, the calf muscles will quickly adapt to that shortened position and will no longer stretch out on their own. To lengthen the muscle, you could foam roll for up to one minute and then perform a stretch. However, foam rolling once a day will never be enough to actually create the change needed to relieve pressure off the knee because the next day you will be right back in your heeled shoe, and your calves will shorten again. In this case, you may want to plan to foam roll and stretch first thing in the morning, at lunch, and before bed. To maximize the benefit, you would also want to include some strengthening exercises for other muscles around the foot.

The frequency and consistency with which you foam roll will play a big part in the benefits you receive. Always consider what you're asking your body to do most of the time. If you notice that you're in the same position for hours each day, then you may need to devote a few minutes throughout the day to your foam rolling and stretching routine.

Foam rolling provides many benefits. Foam rolling before a workout or other physical activity can help you move better and perform better. It is a great technique to include before, during, and after a workout to increase blood flow, stimulate muscles to work more efficiently, initiate the recovery process, and reduce soreness. Foam rolling may be effective at helping to manage pain by introducing motion and temporarily distracting the nervous system. When applied appropriately, these benefits may be noticeable for days. Foam rolling introduces a new stimulus and therefore should be used consistently so the body can adapt. Our next chapter will introduce and explain how foam rolling can be safely integrated into your everyday life.

Chapter 3

FOAM ROLLING SAFETY

Foam rolling is generally considered safe if you follow a few easy guidelines. The most important asset to have when foam rolling is common sense. For example, if you have an injury, don't push the foam roller on it. Or, if you have been experiencing chronic pain, don't use the foam roller as a method of treatment. Always consult with your physician first if you have an injury or medical condition.

Additionally, there are certain sensitive places on the body such as the front of your neck, the armpit, behind the kneecap, and the abdominal region that shouldn't be rolled. And, it should go without saying but always be careful around the head and neck. Another area of concern is the low back: There may be some value in very specific rolling, but aggressive rolling on a large, hard roller should be avoided.

Lastly, misunderstanding the goal of rolling is one of the most frequent mistakes. There is usually no need to roll on something that is made of steel or hard pipe or has large spikes. Sometimes an object that is denser may be necessary, and something with ridges may feel great, but the goal is never to see how much something can hurt. Individuals who approach foam rolling with this attitude and roll on these types of devices have a misunderstanding of the goal. This chapter will tackle foam rolling safety and cover the principles you need to know to ensure you are safe while rolling.

FOAM ROLLING AND MEDICAL CONTRAINDICATIONS

The origins of foam rolling are rooted in massage. Up to this point, researchers have not specifically determined when users should avoid a foam roller, so most of the information available is from massage therapists and has been adapted for foam rolling. Stull and Elliott (2015) suggested that conditions such as osteoporosis, diabetes, high blood pressure, varicose veins, and pregnancy all warrant extra caution while foam rolling. (There could be other conditions that warrant caution—these are just the most common among the general population.) It's not that someone can't foam roll with these conditions—they would just need to be extra careful. These are what we call "relative contraindications," or conditions that require caution when foam rolling.

Osteoporosis

Osteoporosis is a condition that involves weakening of the bones (see figure 3.1). It occurs in both men and women, but is seen more often in women. Osteoporosis is usually associated with menopause in which a greater rate of bone breakdown occurs relative to bone rebuilding. In most cases, the bones of the spine and neck or the femur weaken more readily than other areas. Whether you should use the foam roller if you have osteoporosis depends on the severity of the condition. For example, in very mild cases, it is safe to roll areas of the body that will not experience much pressure when rolling (such as the upper back, shoulders, upper thigh, or lower leg while standing against a wall). Generally plan to avoid areas along the spine or the thigh and hip, even with mild osteoporosis, as these areas usually experience too much pressure when lying on the roller. Instead, these areas could be safely treated by a clinician, massage therapist, or by using minimal pressure standing and leaning against a wall. As previously mentioned (and will be reiterated in this chapter), if for any reason you are unsure whether to roll, consult a health care provider and, with this condition, ask for a bone density scan before you roll.

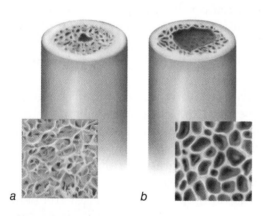

Figure 3.1 Healthy bone *(a)* versus osteoporotic bone *(b)*.

Diabetes

Diabetes in itself is not a contraindication. Rather, it's important to take caution with foam rolling when experiencing some of the systems associated with diabetes. The most notable of symptoms or side effects are diabetic neuropathy, damage to blood vessels, and damage to capillaries. Diabetic neuropathy is a type of nerve damage that may occur in the legs and feet. The symptoms can vary from pain to numbness. The danger with foam rolling areas of neuropathy is that we do not want to cause additional pain. Foam rolling may work to relieve some tension and tightness in muscles, but there is no evidence to suggest it positively affects nerves. Therefore, rolling when there is nerve pain is not recommended. In the case of numbness, the tender spot may not always be obvious. If you were to apply too much pressure to that spot, it could result in bruising or, worse, tissue damage. Over time, high blood sugar causes a hardening of arteries, which can lead to heart attack, stroke, and poor circulation in the lower legs and feet. While there is not much conclusive evidence of the effects of foam rolling on arteries, researchers have suggested there is some effect, as explained in chapter 1. However, when poor circulation is combined with numbness, any bruising caused by foam rolling could set the stage for damage. If circulation is normal, plenty of blood and oxygen is pumped through the lower body, and bruises heal very quickly. When diabetes is present, this healing may not happen as quickly.

Finally, high blood sugar can also thicken the small blood vessels and capillaries. Capillaries are very small and pass blood from the arteries to the veins. One of the most important jobs of the capillaries is to deliver blood and oxygen to organs and carry waste products away from organs. When the walls of the capillaries thicken, they become unable to transmit blood efficiently. In addition, the smaller blood vessels and capillaries may begin to leak. Again, foam rolling has not been shown to have a positive or negative effect. This is a delicate issue that should be addressed by a health care provider before using a foam roller.

High Blood Pressure

When it comes to foam rolling, high blood pressure is one of the more manageable conditions because most people are already managing their high blood pressure with medication. The most important considerations when foam rolling with high blood pressure are body position and breathing. For a few areas of the body that are being rolled (such as the thigh), you may be in a horizontal position. When the heart is level with the rest of the body, this could naturally increase blood pressure—but the increase is usually minimal and foam rolling doesn't usually require you to be horizontal for hours. The other consideration, and likely the most important, is pain. The natural response to pain is to tense up and hold the breath. If you hold your breath, you are simultaneously increasing the amount of pressure in the body, especially if you are also tensing muscles. The combination of holding the breath and tensing the muscles, which you might be doing while foam rolling a painful area, will result in a dramatic increase of pressure on the body and is, therefore, likely to also increase blood pressure. It is important to remember to breathe and relax as much as possible when foam rolling, even if your blood pressure is controlled.

Varicose Veins

Varicose veins are another condition that require caution when foam rolling. Varicose veins are swollen veins that are noticeable under the skin. In most cases, a varicose vein is slightly protruding out of the skin. The lower body is the most common area to experience varicose veins, due to gravity. Veins carry the blood vessels that return deoxygenated blood from around the body to the heart. The heart pumps to drive blood flow and works great when the blood is flowing from the heart down to the extremities. However, blood pressure is lower for blood that is attempting to flow back up toward the heart. Muscle contractions in the legs assist the vessels as they work to push blood back to the heart. To prevent the blood from flowing back down the legs, the body is armed with little valves—essentially blood vessels are one-way streets. However, sometimes the valves weaken, or conditions such as pregnancy could put weight on the vein in the femur, which may inhibit the valves. In these cases, the blood may begin to flow back. This leads to swelling and eventually overall weakening of the vein, which then becomes a varicose vein. If you have varicose veins, foam rolling these weak areas could place too much pressure on them and cause even more damage. So, if you want to foam roll with varicose veins, try to avoid putting pressure directly on the varicose veins. Rolling all around them appears to be safe.

Pregnancy

Pregnancy is another relative contraindication when it comes to foam rolling. Pregnancy affects nearly every system in the woman's body. It can place additional stress on the muscles, bones, and joints; it can even increase metabolism and change the hormones and emotions. Foam rolling during pregnancy could also have a variety of effects. As has been mentioned, foam rolling contraindications are adapted from years of massage therapy findings. The American Congress of Obstetricians and Gynecologists (ACOG), the leading authorities on pregnancy matters, generally advises that if you had been regularly exercising before you became pregnant, then it is safe to continue exercising or to start most types of exercise programs in pregnancy (ACOG, 2016). Exercise does not increase the risk of miscarriage in a normal, low-risk pregnancy. However, it is still highly recommended to discuss any pregnancy exercise routines with a health care provider. The same can be said for massage. Many authorities, such as ACOG and the American Pregnancy Association, highly recommend massage as long as it is relaxing and performed by a therapist who is certified in prenatal massage. Contraindications with massage are typically related to the use of certain types of oils. Some oils, known as emmenagogue essential oils ("emmenagogue" suggests it stimulates blood flow in the pelvic area), may induce uterine contractions. These should not be used in the first trimester, as they may be associated with miscarriage. Foam rolling involves self-application of massage. The user controls the pressure and can, therefore, foam roll to the degree that it is still relaxing. Additionally, foam rolling does not use (nor is it recommended to introduce) any types of oils, so essential oils contraindication does not apply.

Another contraindication with massage and pregnancy is the use of deep techniques. Deep tissue massage is not recommended over the low back

Addressing Pain Safely

Foam rolling is not intended to be used to diagnose or treat any medical condition, including pain. Pain is a complex topic that has yielded volumes of research in past decades. (If you would like to explore this research, read *Explain Pain* by Dr. David Butler and Lorimer Moseley.) It is important to know that pain is an interpretation of an event by the brain, and our feelings of pain are highly subjective. Therefore, sticking any sort of object into an area of pain is never recommended—unless, of course, you have discussed this with your health care provider and have agreed upon this solution.

The areas you choose to roll should be based on a movement assessment, which will be covered in chapter 10. This will give you the best chance of addressing pain or discomfort. Take knee pain, for example. Tendonitis of the knee is very common, and pain is usually felt just above or below the kneecap. This is considered an overuse injury, due to the repetitive loading of the muscles that attach to the kneecap. It might feel instinctive to roll the kneecap if it is hurting, but it will not help. There is no reason to roll the kneecap, and if you do, you may cause additional pain. In order to have any positive influence over this sort of pain, you would most likely need to use the foam roller on the quadriceps and maybe the calf muscles. Research suggest that if these muscles are short, it could lead to overuse of the patellar tendon (attached to the bottom of the kneecap).

Another common issue, especially in active populations, is iliotibial (IT) band syndrome, also known as "runner's knee." In most cases, if someone with runner's knee has a foam roller, they will immediately want to foam roll the IT band. While the knee may feel better after rolling, the pain will come back, usually worse than before. This happens because the IT band isn't doing anything wrong. Contrary to what you may have heard, it does not get tight. It is incapable of such an action. The scientific evidence is very clear on this, and the conclusion is almost always that there is some sort of muscle imbalance at the hip. Therefore, foam rolling the IT band may temporarily help it feel better, but you would still need to address the hip to make a lasting difference. Always assess before you foam roll, and let your movement assessment guide the areas you roll. It is not wrong to roll the IT band, but the foam roller actually has more of an influence on the muscles under the IT band. In most cases, the answer to a physical ailment is not to chase the pain but to find the root cause.

during the first three to four months of pregnancy. Likewise, it is not recommended to deeply massage certain pressure points on the inside of the thigh and calf muscles in the third trimester. Throughout pregnancy, it is important to keep track of blood sugar levels and blood pressure, as an abnormality not only would increase the risk of the pregnancy, but also would be a secondary contraindication for foam rolling. In the third trimester, the hormone relaxin kicks into full gear to relax the muscles around the hips and prepare the body for birth. As the muscles begin to relax, stability may decrease. During this time, foam rolling or release of the fascia around the hips is contraindicated because it may lead to more instability and increase the risk of falling. If you are interested in foam rolling during pregnancy, it is my general recommendation to make sure you are regularly communicating about your training program with your health care provider and always following your physician's orders. While foam rolling is generally safe for the duration of a low-risk pregnancy, it is perfectly fine to cease foam rolling if you begin to feel uncomfortable, can't move into the positions safely, or prefer to see a certified prenatal massage therapist.

COMMON SENSE PRINCIPLES WHEN FOAM ROLLING

In 1764, poet, philosopher, and historian Voltaire quipped, "Common sense is not all that common." This is indeed true when it comes to foam rolling. The following are several common sense principles that may not be that common, especially if you go into your local health club and watch others foam roll!

Once the Tender Spot Is Found, Just Lie There

It seems like foam rolling should be much more fun than just lying still, but often that's what it takes to see the benefit. You do not need to knead the tissue by wiggling side to side, nor should you pump your leg up and down as though you're in step class. You definitely should not attempt to roll as quickly as possible, as though you are on fire. Just lie there and concentrate on your breathing. After a time, you can add in a few very small and very controlled movements (about 1 inch, or 2.5 centimeters, per second). Rolling techniques are covered in Part II.

Only Roll Areas You Know Are Safe

Believe it or not, there are certain sensitive areas of the body that should not be rolled unless the rolling is performed by a physician or therapist. While a licensed and qualified therapist may be able to use their hands to assist, you should not try to roll these areas with an inanimate and unforgiving object such as a baseball.

The Neck

There are certain ways to relax muscles in the upper back and shoulders, but other areas of the neck should be left to the specialists. Do not ever push an object against the front of your neck and, for that matter, I recommend you never even use a foam roller on the sides of the neck. There are two muscles on the side of the neck—the scalene muscle and the sternocleidomastoid muscle—that may be problematic for individuals who sit at computers. They are on each side of the neck, so we have four total. There are also very sensitive nerves and arteries, weaving in, out and around them (see figure 3.2). As these areas can become problematic, leave them for a specialist.

The brachial plexus is a group of nerves that exit the cervical spine, course through the scalene muscles, and provide sensory and motor functions to the entire arm. If the brachial plexus is compressed too much or too frequently, it can be injured—and nervous tissue (nerves) does not repair like muscle tissue. It may be months or even years before it will completely repair itself. The other structure around the neck is the carotid artery, a thick blood vessel around the sternocleido-

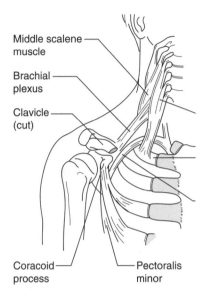

Figure 3.2 Sensitive muscles, nerves, and arteries of the neck.

mastoid that carries blood and oxygen to the brain. While this artery is likely more difficult to damage than the brachial plexus, it is still very sensitive and therefore shouldn't be compressed or stretched too frequently. In this case, using your own hands will allow you to better feel any sensitivities and move away from them if needed. If someone else is working on these areas for you, I highly recommend you ask him or her to avoid using a tool or object. By using your own hands, you will be able to better feel the sensitive structures and get off of them immediately if needed.

The Low Back

There is a good chance that the majority of readers are going to feel sad when they hear this: There is really no reason to use a foam roller on the back, even if it hurts. As previously mentioned, it's better to find the root cause of pain rather than to chase the pain, and that is certainly true for low back pain. Most people with low back are not dealing with a specific low back injury, so the low back itself is not to blame. In the absence of some impact trauma to the low back, the muscles tense up to protect it from more damage. Therefore, jamming a hard object against it is likely to do more harm than good. Foam rolling may temporarily relieve some pain, just like scratching a mosquito bite

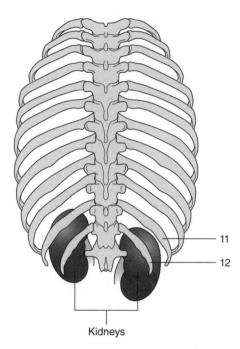

11

12

Kidneys

Figure 3.3 Kidneys and floating ribs in the low back.

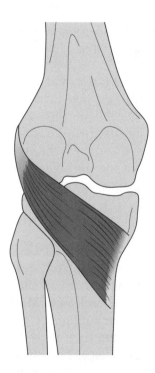

Figure 3.4 Back of the knee.

will temporarily relieve the itch, but it will not fix anything. Also, consider what else could be happening in the area. For example, some individuals initially report low back pain but later discover they have kidney stones. We will cover a simple assessment for the low back in chapter 10; but for now, consider using the foam roller on the muscles of the upper back and around the hips. This is much more likely to reduce the tension felt in the muscles of the low back. In addition, there are some sensitive structures in the area of the low back, such as the kidneys or floating ribs (see figure 3.3), which are unlikely to enjoy direct compression. The kidneys sit just below ribs 11 and 12, which are known as "floating" ribs because they only have one small attachment to the spine and do not connect to the sternum like the other ribs. Although breaking them is unlikely, I would not recommend you apply direct compression to this area (even if you saw something on the Internet or heard a professional tell you it's fine to do). If you are indeed having trouble with the low back, consult with your health care provider or a licensed therapist. Don't just roll on stuff!

The Back of the Knee

Another area that occasionally has some aches and pain is the area behind the kneecap. There are several nerves and arteries in this area, which is known as the "popliteal fossa" because of a muscle called the popliteus. Also in this area is the popliteal artery, the tibial nerve, the common peroneal nerve, and two tiny arteries called the genicular arteries (see figure 3.4). If a popliteal (Baker's) cyst develops at the back of the knee, this should not be rolled (see figure 3.5). A Baker's Cyst is a localized swelling at the back of the knee that is usually caused by overproduction of synovial fluid (a fluid in the joint), often due to arthritis or damage to the knee joint. While a Baker's cyst does not usually lead to any long-term damage,

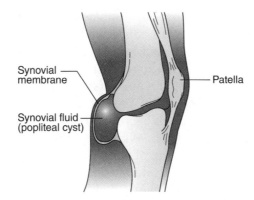

Figure 3.5 Popliteal (Baker's) cyst on the back of the knee.

it often causes sensations of tightness, tension, and pain. The moral of the story here is that there is little reason to foam roll the area behind the knee.

The Groin

On the inside of the thigh is a group of muscles called the adductors. The adductors are five muscles that work to stabilize the hip, among other tasks. However, as you may have guessed from it being in this chapter, you need to proceed with caution. High on the hip, pretty close to the pelvis, is an area known as the "femoral triangle" (see figure 3.6). This is an area of soft tissue, and some important nerves and arteries run through it. The triangle is made up of the inguinal ligament that connects the pubic bone to the iliac crest, the sartorius muscle, and the adductor longus muscle. Inside of this triangle is easy access to the femoral nerve, femoral artery, femoral vein, and the deep inguinal lymph nodes—areas that don't really need to be foam rolled. On the other hand, the adductors are muscles that many people do need to be rolling. So, when rolling this area, proceed with caution and pay attention to anything that feels sensitive. As a general rule of thumb, if you feel a pulse, a zinging pain, numbness, or any unusual pain or sensations, then just maneuver away from the area.

The Hip

Next up on the list of extra sensitive areas is the piriformis, a muscle deep in the

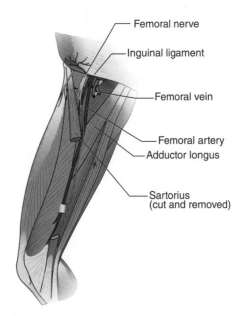

Figure 3.6 The femoral triangle.

hip. This muscle is covered last because, unlike the areas previously mentioned, this is actually an area that most people need to foam roll. But, it is similar to some of the areas around the neck because there is a very important nerve that runs along this area that you do not want to harm. The piriformis is not only a primary rotator of the hip but also has several secondary functions, one of which is hip extension. The gluteus maximus is the muscle that primarily exists to extend the hip, but it often becomes weak and underactive—meaning it simply doesn't want to do its job. When any muscle becomes underactive, our bodies have an amazing system of helpers that kick in. On the other hand, over time this can lead to more dysfunction or injury. In the case of the hip, the piriformis often becomes overworked and, as a result, tenses up. Tension should not be confused with "tightness." Tightness is a sensation; it is not an indication of the length of a muscle. The piriformis is rarely short and tight. Rather, it is usually long and tense.

If the piriformis becomes tense, this can be problematic because there is a large nerve (the sciatic nerve) that runs through or very close to the muscle (see figure 3.7). The sciatic nerve is roughly the thickness of the little finger and is the primary nerve serving the lower extremities. When this nerve is pinched or compressed in the piriformis, you may feel numbness or pain in the buttocks, down the back of the leg, and into the knee. It is important to note, however, that if the sciatic nerve is pinched in the piriformis, the pain will likely not go any lower than the knee.

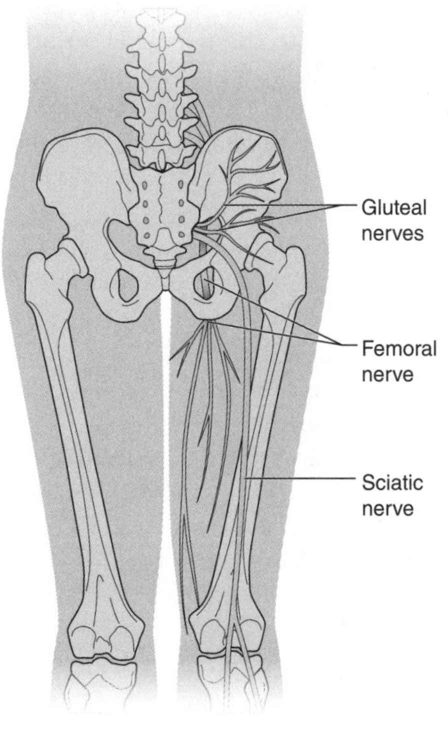

If you have numbness, pain, or tingling down to your foot, this often indicates that the sciatic nerve is being pinched in the spine. If you are unsure about this area, I highly recommend you speak with your health care provider before attempting any of the foam rolling exercises. If it turns out your piriformis is causing the pinching, foam rolling the piriformis may be a great way to relieve some tension. Just refrain from using an incredibly hard and unforgiving object such as a baseball. When the entire body weight is on a small hard object and there is a large important nerve running through the area, it is inadvisable to just lie there forever—approximately one minute is the maximum.

Gluteal nerves

Femoral nerve

Sciatic nerve

Figure 3.7 The sciatic nerve.

The Abdomen

The abdominal region is a sensitive area, but, much like the above regions, it may be rolled with some products and a lot of caution. While it is remote, there is potential to apply too much pressure to organs in the abdominal region. A rough diagram of the abdomen (see figure 3.8) shows everything that could potentially be damaged. Some rolling programs may suggest using a foam roller in this area, but this book will not recommend the use of a foam roller anywhere around the abdomen. It can be safe if done slowly and if on the appropriate product. Still, the safest approach to addressing the abdomen is to consult a licensed therapist or physician.

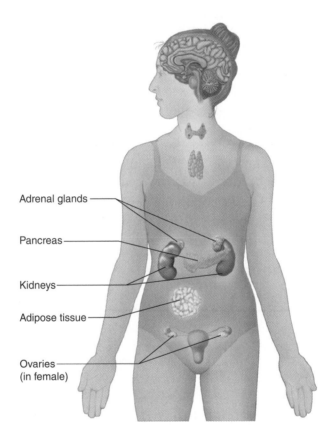

Figure 3.8 Organs of the abdominal region.

Foam rolling is generally a safe practice if you follow some basic principles. The human body is resilient, but the aforementioned sensitive areas need to be approached with caution or completely avoided if you don't feel comfortable.

It's Not About the Pain

It doesn't take long, about .70 seconds, to obtain almost 4 million results about foam rollers on Google (or just "foam" or just "rollers"). Search results suggest some interesting products and recommendations for types of rolling objects, from steel bars and steel rods to rocks, PVC pipe, and random items around the house.

This is befitting of the "cure all" method that was used in medicine for many years. Several hundred, and even thousands, of years ago, whether you were an Egyptian with a migraine or a Greek with a fever, chances were that your doctor would try one particular treatment before all others: bloodletting. Bloodletting is thought to have originated in ancient Egypt and is the process of letting a significant amount of blood, in most cases, drain from the body. Practitioners would cut arteries or veins to let blood out of the body with the thought that it is was ridding the body of disease. The idea is not completely incorrect: As the body loses blood, the body must generate new, healthy blood. However, it wouldn't make a lot of sense to drain the blood to cure a sore throat.

The moral of the story is that we aren't living in the 18th century. We have better research and better products these days. Use a foam roller that is safe and not just a random rod, rock, bar, or piece of steel. Steel and PVC pipe are not made to compress into the body and it could lead to significant tissue damage. The goal is not try to cause more pain but to help your body move better and feel better. Find something that was designed for this process, and purchase one that is made by a company that is doing research to create quality products.

Don't Roll Someone Else

Unless you are a licensed massage therapist or other qualified health care practitioner, don't foam roll your buddy. It seems harmless, but you can understand from all the previously discussed issues that there are many hazards to avoid. Just because it felt good to you doesn't mean it will feel good to a friend, and you won't be able to feel what your friend feels anyway. You could be aggressively smashing the nerves in the neck (or the brachial plexus), and your friend may not know how to tell you to stop or even know that the numbness he or she is feeling in his or her fingers isn't normal.

The most important thing you can do to ensure your safety during foam rolling is to simply remember you don't know it all. It's OK to not always know what is going on with your body. Many health care providers go to college for a minimum of eight years to learn the human body. If you have some sort of condition that you don't understand or are not comfortable foam rolling, speak with one of those highly educated professionals first. The Internet is a great resource, but unfortunately there is such a mix of information that you cannot guarantee what you're reading is right for YOU. Seek help when needed.

Chapter 4

FOAM ROLLING EQUIPMENT

Foam rolling has quickly become one of the fastest growing trends in health, fitness, sports, and even in several medical industries such as physical therapy. Walk into any health club or physical therapy office and you are likely to see some type of foam rolling device. It may not necessarily be foam, but it will have been designed for the same purpose.

The term "foam rolling" has become associated, and often used interchangeably, with self-myofascial release. However, many effective self-myofascial release devices are made out of molded plastic, wood, or hard rubber. Rollers made from compressed foam simply became the most popular when they were released because it is relatively cheap and easy to use.

This chapter covers some of the most popular devices on the market. While this is thorough, it is not an exhaustive list. But, hopefully, you can apply these thoughts to any type of roller and make an informed decision on the roller best suited to your needs.

MULTI-PATTERN DESIGN FOAM ROLLERS

Multi-pattern design foam rollers, as shown in figure 4.1, is one of the most (if not the most) popular foam rollers on the market today. It is made with EVA foam and a PVC core for added reinforcement

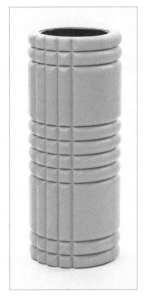

Figure 4.1 Multi-pattern design foam roller.

HISTORY OF ROLLING DEVICES

As has been mentioned in this book a few times, foam rolling began as a method to mimic massage. It is important to reiterate this because when it comes to practical application, you should think like a massage therapist and also remember the roots of the practice have been around for a very long time. While this will not suffice as an exact history of foam rolling, I have taken the time to research U.S. patents on massage rolling devices (see figure 4.2).

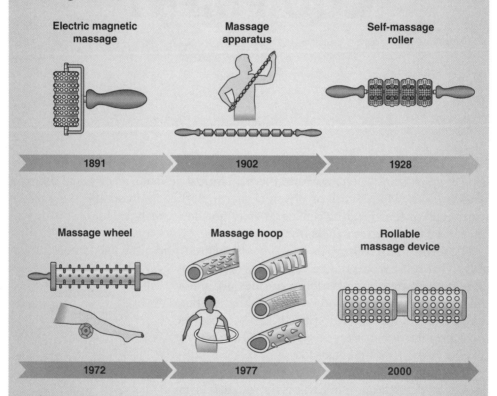

Figure 4.2 History of foam rollers.

On top of all these official-looking patents, I have personally met more than a handful of clinicians and therapists who claim to have used "foam" rolling devices for more than 40 years. In one instance, a rather vocal and vibrant doctor of physical therapy explained to me that in the 1970s, she would cut off contoured wooden table legs and give them to her patients to roll on. Fortunately, these days you don't have to use wooden table legs. A foam rolling industry has developed to offer athletes, health enthusiasts, doctors, and everyone in between a foam roller that fits their budget, is easy to use, and is effective.

and durability. This type of roller is usually available in various sizes, up to 36 inches, or .9 meters, all the way down to about 6 inches, or 15.2 centimeters. The most popular usually falls somewhere in the middle. The various sizes are really a matter of personal preference. The longer rollers are often more comfortable to those who are just beginning a foam rolling program and need extra stability. The medium-sized roller is great for individual use. Many people purchase these rollers to take to the health club with them. They fit nicely into a gym bag and even carry-on luggage for traveling by airplane. This feature does have some consequences, however, because they have been known to disappear off of the gym floor.

The multidimensional pattern on the foam roller is one of the first to be introduced into the market. Almost every foam roller today is available with some sort of a design. The foam is all the same density, but the different sizes of the sections apply a different amount of pressure into the body. This design was sort of a forethought that was later semi-supported by research. The Grid was released in 2006 and later, in 2008, researchers Curran, Fiore, and Crisco found that a foam roller with different surfaces was more beneficial than a regular, smooth roller. This research has not yet been replicated on these type of foam rollers, but there have been several instances where individuals have simply been asked how it feels compared to a regular roller. At the time of this writing, research currently being conducted at a major U.S. university suggests that the grid patterns "just feel better" than other rollers.

HARDER-DENSITY FOAM ROLLERS

Harder-density foam rollers, as shown in figure 4.3, often have a similar design to softer rollers and are a suitable progression from softer foam rollers. The increased density means that the foam roller should influence more layers of tissue with the same amount of compression. Use of this roller is usually not the best way to be introduced to foam rolling though, because it could be too uncomfortable at the outset. It is very difficult to turn foam rolling into a habit if you never want to use the foam roller. In addition, these type of rollers may prove to be a little too intense for certain body parts. For example, rolling the outside of the leg (iliotibial band) may hurt too badly. It is fine to have a small selection of rollers for different body parts, if you choose.

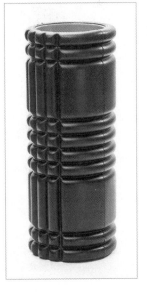

Figure 4.3 Harder-density foam roller.

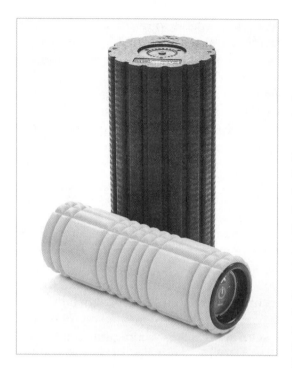

Figure 4.4 Vibration technology foam rollers.

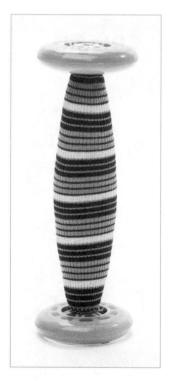

Figure 4.5 Smaller, denser roller.

VIBRATION TECHNOLOGY FOAM ROLLERS

Vibration technology has recently been introduced into foam rollers (see figure 4.4). Vibration helps influence the muscle and tissue in a slightly different manner. Many of these rollers have multiple speeds to accomplish different goals. Lower frequencies tend to have a relaxation effect while higher frequencies have a stimulatory effect. I have performed some very rudimentary research and found that several of these rollers fall within range of all frequencies. The only drawback is the price tag: Unless you can find it on sale somewhere, these rollers generally retail for $99 to $199. Of course, it is important to understand that a significant amount of money and time has been spent on research and development of this foam roller. So, if you can afford the roller, you can be sure you are getting a quality product with sound research.

SMALLER, DENSER ROLLERS

If I had to pick one tool that is easy to use, effective, and portable, I am likely to go with the roller shown in figure 4.5. Many of these rollers are constructed with a steel rod down the center and wrapped with a special material that gives the roller some give. This is an important feature that all foam rolling products need to have.

When compressed into the muscle, rollers should slowly allow a slight bit of conformity around the muscle. While rolling and going through the specific program included in this book, this roller will help to better mobilize and loosen the specific muscle. In addition, this roller is relatively close to the ground, unlike most other rollers that have a diameter of 5 to 7 inches, or 12.7 to 17.8 centimeters. So when rolling the more tender areas of the quadriceps, for example, you can actually lie down to better relax or reduce some of the pressure on the roller.

MASSAGE BALLS

Another highly effective tool is the massage ball (see figure 4.6). These come in a variety of sizes and densities to fit almost anyone. As with any type of roller, the different densities will influence different layers of tissue. A massage ball that is harder will work deeper. It could be used as a progression from a softer roller or in an effort to reach body parts that are harder to access. As noted previously, it is important to recognize that the proper massage ball should allow some conformity. This will ensure better results with the muscles and fascia and decrease the chances of applying too much pressure directly to surrounding nerves. Many times individuals use lacrosse or golf balls for rolling, but it's important to recognize that their density is much harder. As density increases and size decreases, the amount of pressure applied directly to one spot significantly goes up. Additionally, rollers that have no flexibility can be unforgiving. Thus, while rolling with sporting goods equipment may work, the risk of injury increases.

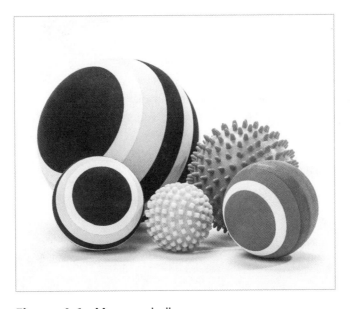

Figure 4.6 Massage balls.

MASSAGE STICKS

Massage sticks are handheld rollers designed to be used by applying pressure to the upper body. Similar to other types of rollers, they are available in different densities and designs to best accommodate each individual.

One common style, as shown in figure 4.7, is constructed with a solid piece of foam and a solid steel rod at the center. The solid piece of foam allows for specific techniques, such as pinning and dragging, that are not as easily performed with handheld rollers that have multiple piece designs. In addition, the handle is called an "Acugrip" and initially appears to be a simple ergonomic design. However, this handle was actually molded after a human thumb. This "point" is great for more targeted work and allows you to safely apply direct compression to problematic muscles. The handle is also made from a stickier type of rubber, which makes it an incredibly valuable piece of the roller. The sticky allows the roller to grip the tissue better. This allows someone to perform techniques more consistent with myofascial release, such as dragging.

Another common massage stick design is constructed with individual rolling pieces and a rod that bends around the muscle, which allows it to apply pressure evenly (see figure 4.8). While I have never seen research supporting this,

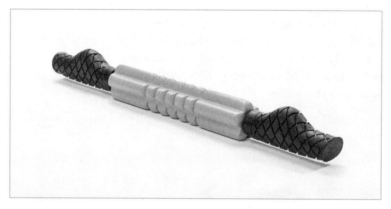

Figure 4.7   Ergonomic massage stick.

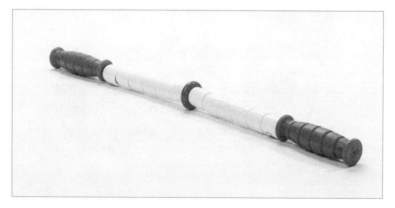

Figure 4.8   Bendable massage stick.

it is a great idea. (The only downside I have experienced with these multiple pieces of plastic was when a bit of my leg hair was pinched in between them.) The massage stick bends when you use upper body strength and allows equal pressure to be applied to the muscle. Although it is not rigid, it is very durable. If you were to break or permanently bend one of these, there is a good chance you were trying to do something you shouldn't have been doing.

Another popular massage stick design is shown in figure 4.9. This roller has a no-bend design and one continuous piece at the center. It is constructed from a softer foam but still allows for some dragging motions to be performed.

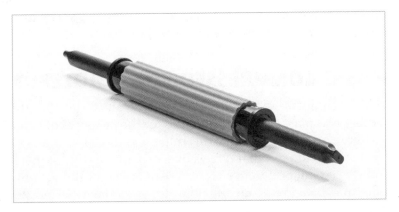

Figure 4.9 Nonbendable massage stick.

DEEP-TISSUE ROLLERS

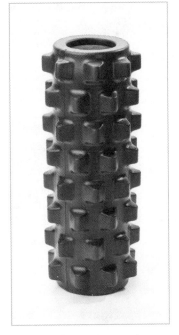

Many people like their foam roller to work deep. These types of rollers have high-profile bumps or nodules on the surface (see figure 4.10). The issue with this type of roller, however, is that the majority of users don't understand what to do with it. Often, these rollers come with extensive educational manuals to teach you how to use them correctly.

These rollers can get very deep and work great if you use it correctly—meaning you are slow and systematic when rolling, working to identify the tissue restrictions and then releasing them. This type of roller works well on the meatier areas of your body that frequently have problematic muscles underneath. Two key spots are the calf muscles and the gluteal muscles. When using it however, you can't just roll up and down at whatever speed you wish. You must slowly roll, repositioning frequently, to get the high-profile

Figure 4.10 Deep-tissue foam roller.

bumps where you want. Then, once you find that "ah-ha" spot, you need to just lie there and relax.

The last thing that must be taken into consideration if your roller has high-profile bumps is the amount of muscle and tissue that is missed when rolling. An important part of foam rolling is to identify knots, adhesions, and trigger points and hold pressure on them. In some cases, these adhesions may be millimeters apart from each other or in some obscure part of the muscle. All of that open space means that if you don't know exactly where to put one of those bumps, then you are likely to miss an enormous amount of tissue. The space missed may be where the problem lies. My suggestion is to at least begin with a flatter device, to search the entire area. After the little knots and adhesions are addressed, then you are free to move on to something that works deeper.

BASIC COMPRESSED FOAM ROLLERS

The "old school" compressed foam roller is where it all started. It is the original foam roller that was mass produced and sold for the purposes of actually foam rolling (see figure 4.11). It seems like this roller was modeled after a swimming pool noodle because that is what it feels like. As with all rollers, there are pros and cons, and personal preference is the most important thing. However, this type of roller may be a great starting point for someone who has never foam rolled before. The downside is that if this is the only roller you have, you will soon adapt to it and need to invest in something else. The other downside is that if multiple people are using it, it will wear down and become flimsy and dirty quickly. In many cases these rollers have to be replaced on a monthly basis. They are available in multiple sizes, can be easily cut to a specific size if you desire, and are super cheap.

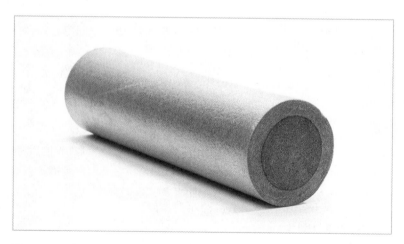

Figure 4.11 Basic compressed foam roller.

Maximizing Comfort When You Foam Roll

Foam rolling in itself is a little uncomfortable, so I suggest you attempt to maximize comfort by performing the rolling on a mat. This could be personal preference, but I suggest avoiding a mat that is too thick. Remember, most foam rolling will take place on the ground and will require you to lie across the roller. If you are on too soft of a surface, the roller will likely sink into the mat and apply less pressure against your body. I suggest you use an everyday yoga mat. These are usually an appropriate thickness and have a grip to them, which will give you a great advantage while foam rolling.

At the end of the day, it really just depends on your preference. The reason there are so many different types of rollers out there is that everyone's needs are different. Get out there and try some before you buy. You can find foam rollers at almost any exercise equipment store, sporting goods store, Target, Walmart, and many specialty stores such as running stores and cycling shops. The product does make a difference but not as big of a difference as how well you use them. While you are out there, don't forget to pick up a relatively thin mat.

Part II

TECHNIQUES

Chapter 5

FOOT AND LOWER LEG

The foot and lower leg are two of the most important areas of the human body. The foot serves as the foundation or platform for everything above it. Anyone who has ever suffered from a painful condition in the foot or ankle likely knows how much it can influence the function of the rest of the body. Foot pain and injuries affect more than 2 million people per year in the U.S. (Martin et al., 2014). Additionally, Cooke and colleagues (2003) suggested that there are approximately 5,600 ankle sprains that are treated in an emergency room per day in the U.K. The muscles of the lower leg have a close relationship with the entire body. The calf muscles attach in or on the foot and some of them travel all the across the knee joint. This means that they can affect both the ankle and the knee. What you also must consider is that the body is continuously trying to maintain its center of gravity over the base of support. The feet are the base of the support, so if the feet and ankles do not move well, the rest of the body will follow in their path.

FOOT

Foam rolling the foot can provide significant relief to tired and achy feet. In addition, foam rolling may also help the entire body move better. In fact, researcher Rob Grieve and colleagues (2015) found that self-myofascial release in the form of foam rolling on the foot could increase flexibility in the hamstrings and low back. This indicates that the foot indeed has major influence over the rest of the body. To better understand how to use the foam roller on the foot, you must first gain an understanding of the foot itself.

Basic Anatomy of the Foot

The foot is composed of a complex set of bones and joints that bear the weight of the entire body while performing movements such as walking, running, jumping, and most other movements. There are 26 bones, approximately 33 joints, and 20 small muscles essentially isolated to the foot, and more than 100 muscles and ligaments that have some sort of influence on the movement of the foot. While all of the moving parts of the foot are important, this book will target the section in the midfoot (see figure 5.1). This is where many of the muscles attach to help support the arch and where foam rolling will likely have the best influence.

Given that the body has approximately 600 muscles and 1/6 of those muscles have either direct or indirect involvement with the foot, it is easy to see the importance of this area. In addition, the foot has thick layers of connective tissue (plantar fascia), blood vessels, and between 100,000 and 200,000 nerves, as estimated by some researchers. All of these structures make the foot susceptible to injury; they also increase the chances that a foot problem will lead to a knee problem, possibly low back pain, and in some cases even neck and shoulder tightness.

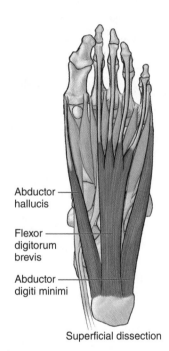

Abductor hallucis

Flexor digitorum brevis

Abductor digiti minimi

Superficial dissection

Figure 5.1 Muscles of the midfoot.

Function of the Foot

The foot is strategically designed to be not only flexible enough for impact but also strong enough to stiffen, thereby becoming a lever to help push off while walking or running. Professor Donald Neumann (2010) suggests that a healthy foot also provides protection and feedback to all the muscles of the lower body. The foot has built-in support, which uses the natural curvature and structure of the foot to absorb impact, all while stabilizing the rest of the body. The foot is capable of an almost incalculable number of different motions. If this incalculable number alone was not large enough, we also have to consider that joints can move in different planes of motion, allowing us to walk up and down hills with varying inclines, run, land from a jump, and help the rest of the body respond to different movements effectively. As biomechanist Katy Bowman (2011) says, "To the foot, the world is flat." In order for the body to feel healthy and move well, the foot must function optimally.

Pros and Cons of Rolling the Foot

There are many reasons to roll the foot as well as several reasons why you should not roll the foot. If you are managing a medical condition, speak with a health care provider before beginning a foam rolling program.

Generally speaking, the foot is a great area to roll when there is general discomfort after a long day or if the foot has been crammed into a high-heeled shoe with a pointy toe. Many shoes force the foot to conform to one particular position without allowing it to move or be stimulated by the ground (yes, your feet actually love the feeling of grass and dirt). That does not mean everyone needs to run barefoot (and most humans shouldn't run entirely barefoot), but rolling the foot before and after cramming it into a shoe may be a lifesaver.

On the other end of the spectrum are the conditions where foam rolling may not be beneficial. Number one on the list is plantar fasciitis. Plantar fasciitis is a debilitating condition causing sharp heel pain and accounts for more than one million doctor visits per year. Like most injuries, plantar fasciitis is classified as an overuse injury—that is, for some reason the connective tissue in the bottom of the foot (plantar fascia) has been repetitively stressed to the point of becoming irritated and painful. This condition can be caused by everything from simply having tight muscles around the ankle to issues rooted in the muscles near the hips. In medicine, "-itis" implies diseases characterized by inflammation. So, the question becomes this: Should you roll your foot when it is already irritated and inflamed? There is no clear answer, but it likely depends on what you are going to roll it with. If you have a medical diagnosis of plantar fasciitis, I would say you should not roll the foot with a golf ball, lacrosse ball, or anything small and hard. If the foot is already irritated, why would you want to jam something into it? That is just going to make it hurt worse.

However, if your approach is to foam roll with something more forgiving, such as a larger or softer roller, then I say go ahead. A softer or larger roller will help to increase fluid flow and possibly help to manage the pain. One of the reasons plantar fasciitis is painful when you first wake up is that fluid has accumulated overnight. Therefore, some light rolling, maybe before even getting out of bed, can be beneficial.

Foam Rolling Techniques for the Foot

To begin, slowly roll the area about 1 inch, or 2.5 centimeters, per second to identify any tender spots. A tender spot is something you identify as being painful or uncomfortable. As a general rule of thumb, on a scale of 1 (no pain) to 10 (worst pain imaginable), search for a spot that feels somewhere between a 5 and an 8. Less than a 5 may not be enough discomfort to encourage change, and any spots with pain greater than an 8 may involve too much pain to allow change. These tender spots may indicate that some type of adhesion, knot, or trigger point is present.

Once a spot is identified, relax the muscle that is being rolled and simply breathe into it. This should generally last for 30 to 60 seconds or until you feel a reduction in tenderness. Then, move on to some small additional motions. While each of these additional motions will be different depending on the body part being rolled, most will follow the same pattern of trying to "pin and stretch" the muscle. You can pin and stretch by holding pressure and moving a joint close to the roller. Never roll up and down as quickly as possible.

BOTTOM OF FOOT WITH MASSAGE BALL

Using a massage ball on the bottom of the foot can allow you to be more specific, as the ball will apply more pressure to one spot, versus a regular foam roller that will apply less pressure to a larger area. The smaller area targets small bones and muscles of the midfoot more directly. However, if you have sensitive feet, have been diagnosed with a foot condition, or are just getting started foam rolling, a larger roller is a better place to start. The firmness of the ball will vary per person. For more intensity, use a harder ball; for less intensity, use a softer ball. One of the easy things about rolling the foot is that you can easily control the amount of body weight applied. In other words, if you use something hard, you can just apply less pressure. I do suggest getting a massage ball made for the foot over using something like a golf ball. It may cost slightly more but will be worth it in the end. For size, look for something between 1.5 and 2.5 inches, or 3.8 and 6.4 centimeters, in diameter.

Begin by placing the massage ball on a smooth surface. You can perform this technique either standing or sitting, but sitting is usually more comfortable and makes it easier to control the amount of pressure on the ball. Place the foot over the massage ball with the massage ball just behind the ball of the foot. The massage ball should be positioned on the inside of the foot to start. Then, slowly roll the foot forward about 1 inch, or 2.5 centimeters, per second, so the massage ball is rolling toward the heel (see figure 5.2a). If you feel a tender spot, stop and hold pressure on it for about 30 seconds or until the tenderness reduces. Do not roll over the heel, rather just up to the front of the heel. Then, slowly roll back the other way. Repeat the process of slowly rolling back and forth about four times. After the fourth roll, position the massage ball near the toe (the starting position) and perform four toe extensions by raising the toes as high as you can and then lowering back down (see figure 5.2b). Next, position the massage ball in the center, just behind the ball of the foot. Repeat the process of slowly rolling forward and back four times, along with the toe extensions. Finally, position the massage ball toward the outside, just behind the ball of the foot, and repeat the process.

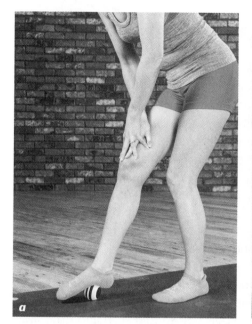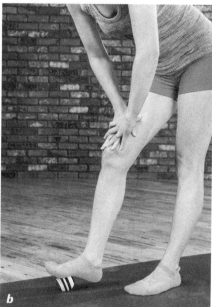

Figure 5.2 Bottom of foot with massage ball: Roll forward and backward *(a)*, and flex toes up and down *(b)*.

BOTTOM OF FOOT WITH FOAM ROLLER

A foam roller is a great tool to use at the beginning if a massage ball is unavailable or is too intense. The larger diameter of the foam roller works the muscles and connective tissue closer to the surface of the skin, instead of working deep. This superficial approach to foam rolling is great if you have a foot injury. With many foot conditions, the goal may be to increase blood flow and not release deep tissue. A regular foam roller can accomplish this purpose and is likely to provide a quick reduction of discomfort.

Begin by placing the foam roller on a smooth surface. You can perform this technique either standing or sitting, but sitting is usually more comfortable and makes it easier to control the amount of pressure. Place the foot over the foam roller, with the roller just behind the ball of the foot. The foam roller will be large enough to cover most of the area you are rolling. Therefore, the rolling will involve small motions. Slowly roll the foot forward about 1 inch, or 2.5 centimeters, per second, so the foam roller is rolling toward the heel (see figure 5.3a). If you feel a tender spot, you should stop and hold pressure on it for about 30 seconds or until the tenderness reduces. Do not roll over the heel, rather just up to the front of the heel. Then, slowly roll back the other way. Repeat the process of slowly rolling back and forth about four times. After the fourth roll, position the foam roller where it is near the toe (the starting position) and perform four pivot motions of the foot by simply twisting the foot side-to-side (see figure 5.3b). Because the roller covers so much area, you only need to repeat this rolling and twisting two times.

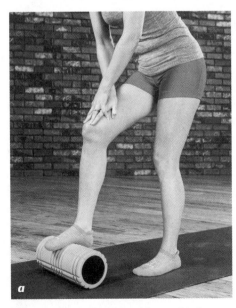
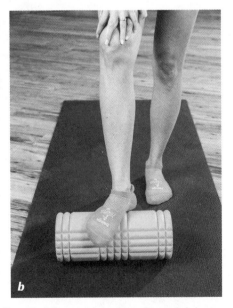

Figure 5.3　Bottom of foot with foam roller: Roll forward and backward (a), and twist side-to-side (b).

LOWER LEG

The foot is an important part of the body and has a significant impact on how the body feels and performs. However, many of the muscles that control the foot are located in the lower leg. The muscles of the calves, for example, connect to the body of the foot through connective tissue. Therefore, if the muscles in the lower leg do not function optimally, then the foot—and the rest of the body—may pay the price.

Basic Anatomy of the Lower Leg

The lower leg is simply the area between the knee and the ankle. For foam rolling purposes, this book will discuss the calf muscles that extend through the back of the lower leg and the outside of the lower leg (the fibularis, or peroneus muscles). This whole area of the body is frequently under a significant amount of stress and tension.

The muscles in the back of the lower leg are commonly referred to as the calves, although other muscles are located there as well (see figure 5.4). The muscles of the lower leg are divided into two different compartments: deep and superficial. The deep compartment contains muscles that are closer to the bone; as you could likely guess, the superficial compartment contains the muscles that are closer to the skin.

The deep compartment contains the tibialis posterior muscle, the flexor hallucis longus muscle, the flexor digitorum longus muscle, and the flexor hallucis brevis muscle. You likely do not need to remember these muscle names, but you should remember that most of these muscles connect to the toes. Therefore, when you foam roll the lower leg, you can influence and positively affect the foot. The superficial compartment contains the gastrocnemius muscle and soleus muscle. Again, you likely do not need to remember the names, but you should know that these muscles do not attach to toes. However, they do attach to the foot. The gastrocnemius and soleus attach to a very thick tendon known as the Achilles tendon. The Achilles tendon is one of the thickest and most powerful bundles of connective tissue in the body. It attaches to the heel bone and surrounding plantar fascia (connective tissue on the bottom of the foot) as well as the two calf muscles. The Achilles is said to be the most important factor in a human's ability to maintain a running gait. The thick interaction of collagen, which receives little blood flow, makes this area of the body very resistant to deformation, which allows it to better store energy. However, due to the lack of blood flow, if the Achilles becomes a problem and you develop a condition such as Achilles tendinitis, it can be very difficult to treat. Therefore, foam rolling the lower leg may help to maintain adequate blood and fluid flow, preventing Achilles problems from developing.

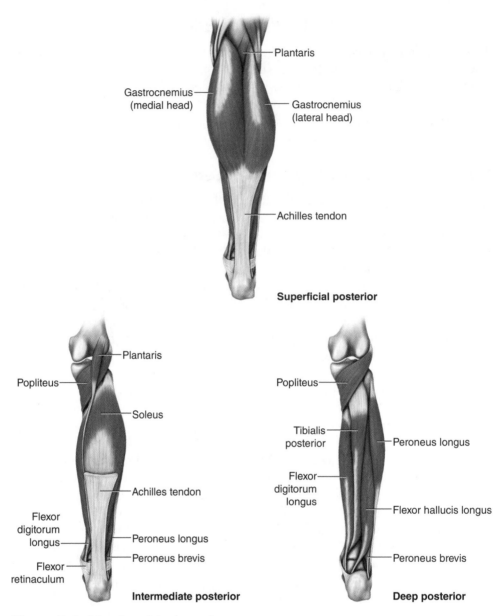

Figure 5.4 Muscles of the lower leg.

Function of the Lower Leg

The lower leg functions as a propulsive mechanism. The muscles in this area attach to the foot and many go above the knee. They help to point the toes, and this movement works as a lever to move the body up and forward. The muscles in the lower leg have both high endurance and normally a good amount of power. Therefore, they also help to maintain proper posture. If these muscles are able to lengthen and shorten optimally, they can help increase performance and decrease the chance of injury.

Similar to the foot, the types of shoes we wear, the position of the ankle, and even how we walk can affect these muscles. Consider the person who appears to drag or waddle when walking. The body is made to use the powerful gluteals to extend the hip while the powerful quadriceps extend the knee and the calves extend the ankle. Together these muscles not only move the body forward but also send the body upward. We walk this way, moving up and down, in order to store elastic energy in the muscles and other connective tissue, thereby making walking incredibly efficient. However, if you waddle when you walk, the gluteus maximus cannot do its job and the other muscles end up doing more than intended: The calf muscles have to work harder, and the whole lower leg is put in a less than ideal position. It is very likely that this exacerbates or even causes many conditions such as plantar fasciitis or ankle sprains. Over time, these muscles shorten, which leads to even worse mechanics and problems. In order to move correctly, the ankle must flex, allowing the knee to move forward and the rest of the body to travel efficiently.

Pros and Cons of Rolling the Lower Leg

The muscles of the lower leg influence the movement of the ankle. The ankle is one of the largest joints closest to the ground; if it doesn't move correctly, much of the upper body will also have a difficult time moving. In modern society, many people do not walk with the feet straight, as the feet are designed to do. When the feet are straight, the body can naturally stabilize and properly support the foot and lower leg. However, if the calf muscles have lost their ability to extend properly, then the foot must compensate. Often, it does so by flattening. Of course, some people have feet that are structurally flat, meaning the bones do not support an arch. However, most people actually have a mechanical flat foot, meaning the muscles are causing or allowing the flattening. Oddly enough, the calf muscles may be to blame.

Short calf muscles may also contribute to issues such as low back pain. When we perform everyday motions, such as squatting, the ankle, knee, and hip should all move together. This allows the muscles that should be doing the work to actually do the work; it also allows the muscles that should not be working to relax or stabilize. However, if the ankles don't move correctly, this alters the entire motion, abnormally loading areas such as the low back. So, foam rolling the muscles of the lower leg may help to reduce or prevent low back pain.

Of course, there may also be times when the lower leg should not be rolled. If you have varicose veins, you can still roll, but you should proceed with caution. As explained in chapter 3, it is generally inadvisable to roll directly on varicose veins, but you could try to roll around them. In addition, be very careful with diabetes that has escalated and introduced visible swelling of the lower leg. In some cases, some light massage may be indicated, but, as always, speak to a health care provider before you begin.

Foam Rolling Techniques for the Lower Leg

To begin, slowly roll the area, about 1 inch, or 2.5 centimeters, per second, to identify any tender spots. A tender spot is something you identify as painful or uncomfortable. As a general rule of thumb, on a scale of 1 (no pain) to 10 (worst pain imaginable), search for a spot that feels somewhere between a 5 and an 8. Less than a 5 may not be enough discomfort to encourage change, and any spots with pain greater than an 8 may involve too much pain to allow change. These tender spots may indicate that some type of adhesion, knot, or trigger point is present.

Once a spot is identified, relax the muscle that is being rolled and simply breathe into it. This should generally last for 30 to 60 seconds or until you feel a reduction in tenderness; then, begin to add small motions. While each of these additional motions will differ depending on the body part being rolled, most will follow the same pattern of trying to "pin and stretch" the muscle. You can do this by holding pressure and moving a joint close to the roller. Never roll up and down as quickly as possible.

POSTERIOR LOWER LEG WITH FOAM ROLLER

Unlike the foot, it is more challenging to control the amount of pressure on the roller when foam rolling the calves. Therefore, I suggest you begin with a larger, softer roller and progress to something harder overtime. Using a foam roller on the lower leg will target all of the muscles mentioned in this section. If you recall, the muscles are essentially divided into two compartments: one closer to the surface and the other deeper. While the compression from the regular foam roller will help the surface muscles more, all of the muscles in the calf region will experience the benefits. I suggest everyone roll their calves. They appear to be short and tight in the majority of individuals, whether you are having knee pain or even neck tension. If you spend a few minutes on the calves almost every day, it will improve how you move and reduce many nagging aches.

Begin by sitting on a comfortable surface. The floor usually works well. However, if you can't get on the floor, then feel free to use two chairs side by side or a bench. Place one of your legs on the roller, with the roller positioned just above the ankle. If you prefer more pressure, then cross the opposite leg over the top. If this is too much pressure, uncross the legs. Keep the feet relaxed as you roll. Your hands should be positioned slightly behind the hips with your fingers pointed away from the body. To roll, you will need to lift your hips off the floor. They don't need to be high off the floor, but enough so you can move your body forward. Raise the hips and begin to slowly roll forward about 1 inch, or 2.5 centimeters, per second (see figure 5.5a). Remember if you find a tender spot, stop and hold for about 30 seconds. As you hold, feel free to set the hips down on the floor, but maintain the pressure from the other leg. After the tenderness is reduced, slowly roll up and down the muscle about four times. Then, position the roller near the center of the lower leg and perform four side-to-side motions of the leg (see figure 5.5b). Together these motions will reduce the tension and add movement back into the area.

If you feel as though you need more pressure, or if you have been working on this for a few weeks, you can progress by performing the same technique on a smaller or harder foam roller. If the roller covers less surface area, it will put more direct pressure on the deeper muscles. Likewise, a harder roller will also help you reach the deeper muscles. That said, remember that reaching deep into the muscles doesn't always need to be the goal. Use the density and size that is uncomfortable but that doesn't cause too much pain.

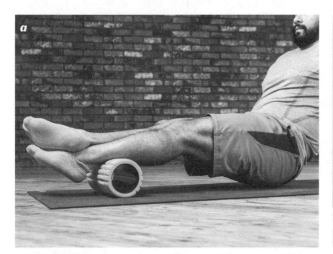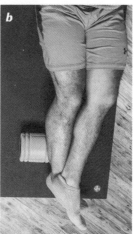

Figure 5.5 Posterior lower leg with foam roller: Roll forward and back (a) and side to side (b).

OUTSIDE LOWER LEG EXERCISE I

To target the muscles on the outside of the lower leg, choose the size of foam roller that suits you best. The muscles you will target with this exercise are not as thick as the calf muscles, but it is also harder to achieve the same amount of pressure that you could achieve on the calves. Therefore, you may want to try both a larger, softer roller and a smaller, harder roller to see which you prefer. It is important to address the entire outside of the lower leg. Muscles near both the ankle and the knee may be problematic. If you have chronic ankle sprains or even knee pain, you will benefit from rolling these muscles as it reduces tension and restores normal movement in the ankle and knee.

Begin by sitting on a comfortable surface. The leg to be rolled should be placed in front of you, with the hip rotated out so the outside of the leg can be flat on the ground. Place the leg on top of the roller and position the roller near the ankle. If you need additional pressure, use an arm to press down. Slowly begin rolling by moving the leg down a few inches or centimeters (see figure 5.6a). If you find a tender spot, hold pressure for about 30 seconds. If there are no tender spots, roll back up to the ankle. Work this area just 3 to 4 inches, or 7.6 to 10.2 centimeters, at a time; rolling the whole thing can be tricky in this position. Roll each section about four times, moving 1 inch, or 2.5 centimeters, per second. After rolling this section four times, perform cross-frictions by moving the leg side to side over the roller (see figure 5.6b). In a cross-friction, the roller will grip the clothing or skin and create a shearing force in the area. This is a great technique to work the fascia. Repeat this process a few inches at a time all the way up the outside of the lower leg. Work all the way to just below the knee.

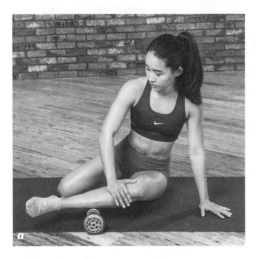 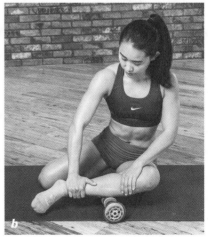

Figure 5.6   Outside lower leg I: Roll forward and back *(a)* and side to side *(b)*.

OUTSIDE LOWER LEG EXERCISE II

If you'd like to progress the technique for the outside of the lower leg, move on to this exercise, which can be performed on the same roller but uses a different body position. The position will place significantly more pressure on the roller and, if performed correctly, will use the core muscles to stabilize the body. It is inadvisable to perform this exercise if you do not have at least a foundational level of core strength developed. However, if you do have the strength, this is a great technique to use as part of a warm-up, as it will help loosen up the peroneals and activate the core muscles.

Begin by lying on your side on a smooth, comfortable surface. Next, place the leg over the roller so the outside of the lower leg is touching it. The roller should be positioned just above the ankle. Place your elbow and forearm just below the shoulder, and raise your hips up into a side plank (see figure 5.7). For extra stabilization, you can place the leg that isn't being rolled, as well as the opposite arm, in front of you. If you desire extra pressure, stack your legs on top of each other. To best address this area and make it easier, break the rolling into two separate parts: (1) Roll from the ankle to halfway up the lower leg, and (2) roll from halfway up the lower leg to just below the knee. To begin rolling, move the body down toward the knee (so the roller moves up) at 1 inch, or 2.5 centimeters, per second. If you find a tender spot, hold pressure for about 30 seconds. Roll through the area about four times. Then, reposition the roller halfway up the leg, and repeat the process on the top half of the outside of the lower leg.

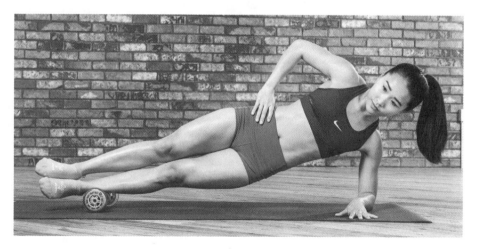

Figure 5.7   Outside lower leg II.

Together the foot and lower leg composes one of the most important areas of the body. Either, or both, of these can contribute to pain and discomfort. Even if your feet or calves aren't hurting, I recommend that you begin your foam rolling program at the foot and lower leg every day. Most of us tend to use and abuse our feet on a daily basis. Giving them some TLC will help your entire body move and feel better.

Chapter 6

UPPER LEG

The upper leg includes the muscles between the knee and pelvis. Many of these muscles cross both the knee and hip joints but can still be generally considered muscles of the upper leg. (Chapter 5 addressed the muscles below the knee joint, and chapter 7 will address the muscles above the hip joint.) For purposes of this discussion, the main muscles that make up the upper leg are the quadriceps, adductors, and hamstrings. Other structures around the upper leg will be discussed here, including the iliotibial (IT) band. When you finish this chapter, you will have a much better understanding of not only how to roll these areas, but also what might be causing dysfunction and tightness.

Here, the muscles of the upper leg will be discussed separately, based on region. However as this is not an exhaustive look at anatomy, and you cannot isolate muscles when you foam roll anyway, this chapter discusses the muscles as they function in a group.

QUADRICEPS

The quadriceps are some of the better understood muscles of the body. They are prominent, easy to see, and generally easy to train. However, there is more to them than is generally considered.

THE ROLE OF THE UPPER LEG IN LOWER BACK PAIN

The common question, "What do the muscles in the legs have to do with low back pain?" does not have an easy answer. Many of the muscles in this chapter attach to the pelvis, which means they have some sort of influence on the position of the pelvis. In many cases, the muscles in the front (quadriceps) pull the hips down, while the muscles in the back (hamstrings) tense to resist the pull from the front. When the pelvis changes its position, the low back (lumbar spine) also changes its position—it is how we are made. When this change in position happens for short periods, it is not a big deal because our bodies are resilient and can repair themselves. However, if the pelvis is in this position day after day, then the muscles of the low back are likely to begin to tighten in response. This is actually very normal and expected when the hips are out of alignment. Most people try to relax the low back muscles with massage that targets the low back, heat therapy, stretches, or over-the-counter pain medicines, without addressing the muscles that attach to the hips. The point is, if you are dealing with low back pain that has worsened and is not related to a specific injury, you probably need to begin looking at other muscles around the hips. This will be further explored in chapter 7.

Basic Anatomy of the Quadriceps

The quadriceps is a muscle group broken into four parts (hence, "quad"), located on the front of the upper leg (see figure 6.1). All four parts cross the knee joint, which means when they contract (shorten), they extend the knee. This also means that when they relax (lengthen), they allow the knee to bend. Closer to the top of the upper leg, three of the four muscles attach to the femur and the fourth muscle crosses the hip joint to attach to the pelvis. If a muscle crosses a joint, then that muscle can create movement around that joint.

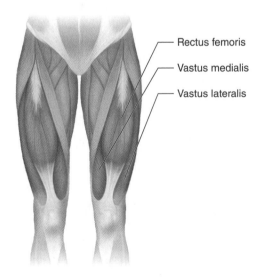

Rectus femoris

Vastus medialis

Vastus lateralis

Figure 6.1 Muscles of the quadriceps.

Therefore, one of the quadriceps, the rectus femoris, can cause the leg to bend at the hip.

When it comes to the muscles as a group, one particular quadriceps muscle is worth noting because it will come up again later in this chapter. The vastus lateralis is the largest of the four muscles and is located on the outside of the leg. This muscle crosses the knee joint to attach to the lower leg through the kneecap but does not cross the hip joint. The size, strength, and position of this muscle gives it massive influence over the lower leg and the knee. In addition, this muscle is located underneath another important structure: the IT band. Remember this as it will come up again later in this chapter.

Function of the Quadriceps

The quadriceps work to extend the knee when shortening and allow the knee to bend when relaxing. If you want to understand the function of the quadriceps, you must consider what happens when the feet are on and off the ground.

An exercise that involves keeping the feet on the ground or in a fixed position is called a "closed-chain exercise," meaning multiple joints have to move. Consider the squat: Squatting requires the ankles, knees, and hips to move in a coordinated fashion, while the feet remain in place. If one of these joints does not move, then a squat is almost impossible. For example, if you were to attempt a squat when the knees couldn't move, you would fall backward. This multi-joint coordination allows the body to maintain its center of gravity over the base of support.

In a squat, the quadriceps can create some interesting motions rarely seen in an anatomy textbook. Consider this: When standing up from a chair, the quadriceps shorten to produce knee extension. However, since the body has an inherent need to maintain the center of gravity, the hips will also extend. The hip muscles will be discussed in detail in chapter 7; for now, it's important to know that if these muscles are not doing their job, then the quadriceps will begin to do more work and eventually take over. On the other hand, anatomy textbooks do generally show that the quadriceps work to extend or straighten the knee when they shorten. As you can see from this brief example, muscles are capable of much more than one motion. The quadriceps are large, powerful, and willing to do all the extra work if necessary.

Pros and Cons of Rolling the Quadriceps

The quadriceps are willing to do a lot of work. They do this because most of them are powerful, single-joint muscles. However, for the body to function properly and optimally, we do not want the quadriceps to do all of the work. They often become overactive and begin doing the work of both the calves and the gluteals. If you want to push the other muscles to get back to doing their job, you must first help the quadriceps to relax. You can do this with massage. However, in between sessions with your massage therapist, the foam roller is a great tool to use daily.

Foam Rolling Techniques for the Quadriceps

To begin, slowly roll the area about 1 inch, or 2.5 centimeters, per second to identify any tender spots. A tender spot is something you identify as painful or uncomfortable. As a general rule of thumb, on a scale of 1 (no pain) to 10 (worst pain imaginable), search for a spot that feels somewhere between a 5 and an 8. Less than a 5 may not be enough discomfort to encourage change, and any spots with pain greater than an 8 may involve too much pain to allow change. These tender spots may indicate that some type of adhesion, knot, or trigger point is present.

Once a spot is identified, relax the muscle that is being rolled and simply breathe into it. This should generally last for 30 to 60 seconds or until you feel a reduction in tenderness; then, add small motions. While each of these additional motions will differ depending on the body part you are rolling, most will follow the same pattern of trying to "pin and stretch" the muscle. You can pin and stretch by holding pressure and moving a joint close to the roller. Never roll up and down as quickly as possible.

QUADRICEPS EXERCISE I

This quadriceps rolling technique is performed on a large, soft roller. Begin with whatever tools you have, but at some point, to continue seeing results, you may need to progress to something either smaller or denser. Since the quadriceps is a larger group of muscles, we divide the muscles into two zones. Zone 1 includes the muscles from the knee to halfway up the leg; Zone 2 includes the muscles from halfway up the leg to the hip. Zone 1 will target all four of the muscles but not necessarily the entire quadriceps. By completing Zone 2, you can ensure that the entire muscle is addressed. If you are dealing with knee pain, be thorough with Zone 1. Rotate the leg in different directions until you find the most tender spot. If you have low back discomfort or hip pain, then put that same focus on Zone 2. The top of Zone 2 will begin to address more of the hip flexor part of the quadriceps. It is vitally important to roll this area if the hips are leading to low back pain. When rolling the quadriceps, you will have a considerable amount of bodyweight on the roller. Therefore, I suggest you begin with a regular-sized roller and slowly progress to a harder or smaller device over time.

Begin in a face-down position on the ground, and place the foam roller near the knee of the leg you are rolling; place the other leg out to the side. Slowly roll by pushing your body down so the roller moves up the leg (see figure 6.2a). When you find a tender spot, hold for about 30 seconds. Then, roll through this area about four times. Next, while keeping the spine neutral, bend and extend the knee four to five times to help stretch out the muscle (see figure 6.2b).

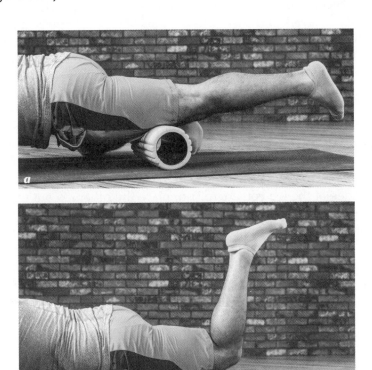

Figure 6.2 Quadriceps I: Roll up and down (a), and bend and extend (b).

QUADRICEPS EXERCISE II

This technique is an additional option for rolling the quadriceps. If you experienced considerable discomfort while performing Quadriceps Exercise I, then there is no need to perform Exercise II. However, if you are experienced with foam rolling and are ready for a progression, move to Quadriceps Exercise II. For this technique, use a smaller diameter and slightly denser roller to influence more layers of tissue.

Since this technique is a form of deep tissue foam rolling, it is best to divide the leg into three zones: Zone 1 will move from the knee to one-third of the way up the leg; Zone 2 will move from one-third to two-thirds of the way up the leg; and Zone 3 will move from two-thirds of the way up the leg to the hip. In each zone, perform steps a, b, and c. This technique will take a little longer than Quadriceps Exercise I. It is common for it to take three to five minutes. If you have a shoulder injury or weak core, this technique will offer a few options to help you successfully complete the foam rolling.

Begin in a face-down position on the ground, and place the foam roller near the knee of the leg you are rolling; place the other leg out to the side. Slowly begin to push yourself down so the roller moves up the leg at 1 inch, or 2.5 centimeters, per second until you find a tender spot (see figure 6.3a). When you find it, hold for about 30 seconds. Then, roll up and down through the muscle about four times. Next, while keeping the spine neutral, move your leg side to side for two complete motions, dragging across the roller to perform a cross-friction (see figure 6.3b). While staying in that same spot, stretch the muscle by bending and extending the knee two times (see figure 6.3c). Once this is complete, perform the same routine slightly higher on the area, remembering to divide the leg into three total zones.

If you have a shoulder injury, or if the shoulders become tired, you can place a support—such as a yoga block or additional foam roller—under the chest or abdomen. This is not intended to support all of your weight but to share the weight with your arms and allow for a more pleasant rolling experience. In addition, if you find a very tender spot, you can safely rest your hips on the ground. This will allow you to breathe and relax better, which will lead to a better result.

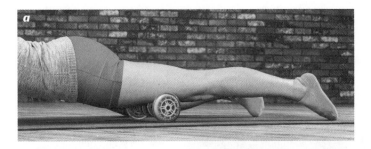

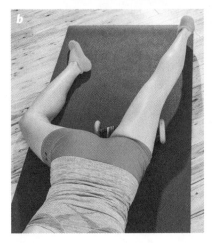
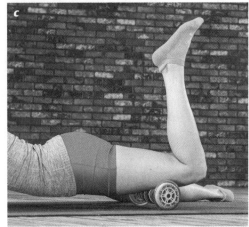

Figure 6.3 Quadriceps II: Roll up and down *(a)* and side to side *(b)*, and then bend and extend *(c)*.

HAMSTRINGS

The hamstrings are muscles on the back of the upper leg. They are often blamed for many problems that they may or may not actually cause. If you gain a better understanding of these muscles, you will be in a better position to assess whether you should roll them.

Basic Anatomy of the Hamstrings

The body has three hamstrings: the semimembranosus, the semitendinosus, and the biceps femoris (see figure 6.4). These muscles are often misunderstood and treated poorly. Hamstrings are multi-joint muscles that cross both the knee and the hips. They find their origin at the bottom of the pelvis on a bone called the ischium. The ischium is also called the "sits bone" because when you are sitting with good posture, this is the bone you should feel on the chair. The hamstrings then run down the back of the leg, cross the knee, and attach to the bone in the lower leg called the tibia.

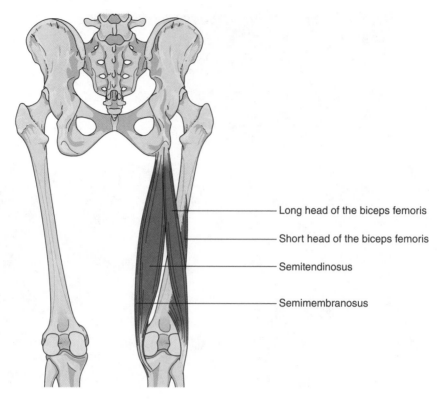

Figure 6.4 Muscles of the hamstrings.

It should be noted that the hamstrings are very different from the quadriceps. The quadriceps are large and powerful single-joint muscles, whereas the hamstrings are not. Most people have much larger quadriceps than hamstrings because their function is very different.

Function of the Hamstrings

The average anatomy textbook will tell you that the hamstrings bend the knee and help extend the hip. That makes sense, since the hamstrings cross both the knee and the hip joint. However, anatomy textbooks generally do not explain that the hamstrings do not perform the majority of knee bending during normal movements. When you walk or run, momentum is doing a significant amount to bend the knee. The hamstrings function more to help extend the hip and, more importantly, stabilize posture. If the center of gravity, which is just behind the belly button, is shifted forward, the hamstrings contract and tighten—a basic stabilization mechanism. Even looking down at a phone, for example, will shift the body forward and require a muscle to contract for support. Often, it is the hamstrings that contract to stabilize the pelvis, thereby offering support for the upper body.

Pros and Cons of Rolling the Hamstrings

For the majority of people in modern society, the hamstrings are not short and tight. Rather, they are long and taut, probably because they are helping to stabilize the pelvis. Imagine a rubber band: If you pull the rubber band, it will lengthen and tighten. Too often, muscle tightness is confused with muscle shortness when it may mean one of several things, such as an irritated nerve. For example, there is a large nerve that runs down the hamstrings (the sciatic nerve). Therefore, you do not need to always foam roll the hamstrings to lengthen them; you may want to roll them to increase blood flow or reduce tension. So, how do you know if the tightness sensation you are feeling is really the hamstrings? You have to perform an assessment and look at posture. This will tell you more about what your hamstrings need.

When foam rolling the hamstrings, you may not feel the same discomfort as with the calves, the quadriceps, or other areas. As explained, they may not actually be short and tight—therefore, they may not be painful. The answer is not to find a way to make it painful by getting on a harder roller or having a friend stand on your leg. Instead, the hamstrings may not need it as much other muscles. Rolling the hamstrings is still valuable if you choose to do it, though, since you can use the technique to increase fluid movement.

Foam Rolling Techniques for the Hamstrings

To begin, slowly roll the area about 1 inch, or 2.5 centimeters, per second to identify any tender spots. A tender spot is something you identify as being painful or uncomfortable. As a general rule of thumb, on a scale of 1 (no pain) to 10 (worst pain imaginable), search for a spot that feels somewhere between a 5 and an 8. Less than a 5 may not be enough discomfort to encourage change, and any spots with pain greater than an 8 may involve too much pain to allow change. These tender spots may indicate that some type of adhesion, knot, or trigger point is present.

Once you identify a spot, relax the muscle that is being rolled and simply breathe into it. This should generally last for 30 to 60 seconds or until you feel a reduction in tenderness; then, add some small motions. While each of these additional motions will be different depending on the body part you are rolling, most will follow the same pattern of trying to "pin and stretch" the muscle. You can do this by holding pressure and moving a joint close to the roller. Never roll up and down as quickly as possible.

HAMSTRINGS WITH FOAM ROLLER

Here, you will also divide the hamstrings up into two zones. Zone 1 involves rolling from the knee to halfway up the leg; Zone 2 involves rolling from halfway up the leg to the hip.

Begin by sitting with your legs in front of the body, and place the foam roller just above the knee on the hamstring. Place your hands near your hips with the fingertips pointed away from the body. Then, raise your hips slightly off the ground and push your body forward so the roller comes up the hamstring (see figure 6.5a). Roll until you find a tender spot, and hold for about 30 seconds. After the time is up, then slowly roll through the muscle four times. Next, move the leg side to side across the roller to perform a cross-friction (see figure 6.5b).

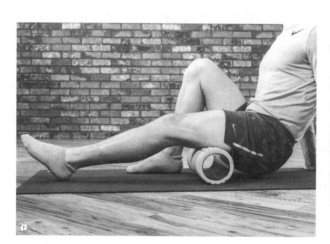
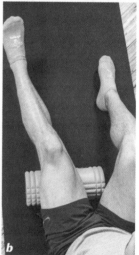

Figure 6.5 Hamstrings with foam roller: Roll forward and back *(a)* and side to side *(b)*.

ADDUCTORS

The adductors are a group of five muscles located on the inside of the upper leg. These muscles can cause as many problems as the large muscles on the front or the stringy muscles on the back.

Basic Anatomy of the Adductors

The adductors include the adductor brevis, adductor longus, adductor magnus, pectineus, and gracilis (see figure 6.6). The muscles are named based on their size and location. The brevis is small, the longus is long, and the magnus is the largest. All adductors attach to the pelvis, so they cross the hip joint (but only the gracilis crosses the knee joint).

Function of the Adductors

As the name implies, the adductors adduct the leg. "Adduction" means bringing together, or moving something closer to the midline of the body. With the muscles positioned on the inside of the upper leg, they can bring the leg to the midline of the body. However, we rarely do this. The body does slightly move the leg toward the midline

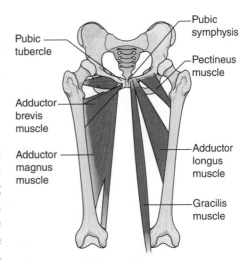

Figure 6.6 Muscles of the adductors.

during walking and running, but it isn't significant. Less commonly known, the adductors also flex and extend the hip. When the hip is bent, as when you are seated in a chair, this is the position of flexion. In the position, the majority of the adductors are shortened. This means that the adductors play a role on the position of the pelvis. Over time, with too much sitting, the adductors become overactive.

Pros and Cons of Rolling the Adductors

For the majority of the population that is relatively sedentary, the adductors become short and problematic. This can pull the pelvis into an anterior pelvic tilt, where the front of the pelvis is dipped forward. Additionally, short adductors pull the knee inward. This is evident when squatting to sit or stand or walking stairs. If the knee moves inward during these motions, it could signify that the adductors need to be foam rolled and probably stretched.

Foam Rolling Techniques for the Adductors

To begin, slowly roll the area about 1 inch, or 2.5 centimeters, per second to identify any tender spots. A tender spot is something you identify as being painful or uncomfortable. As a general rule of thumb, on a scale of 1 (no pain) to 10 (worst pain imaginable), search for a spot that feels somewhere between a 5 and an 8. Less than a 5 may not be enough discomfort to encourage change, and any spots with pain greater than an 8 may involve too much pain to allow change. These tender spots may indicate that some type of adhesion, knot, or trigger point is present.

Once you identify a spot, relax the muscle that is being rolled and simply breathe into it. This should generally last for 30 to 60 seconds or until you feel a reduction in tenderness; then, add some small motions. While each of these additional motions will be different depending on the body part you are rolling, most will follow the same pattern of trying to "pin and stretch" the muscle. You can do this by holding pressure and moving a joint close to the roller. Never roll up and down as quickly as possible.

ADDUCTORS EXERCISE I

Divide the adductor into two zones: Zone 1 involves rolling from the knee to halfway up the leg; Zone 2 involves rolling from halfway up the leg all the way up to the pelvis.

Begin by lying face down, and place the foam roller next to you with its long axis parallel to your body. Then, place the leg you are rolling over the roller. Place your forearms on the ground to support the upper body. The goal of this position is not to perform a plank, but to allow you to move your body side to side comfortably. To roll, slowly shift your body by lifting some pressure off the floor and moving toward the roller so the roller moves up the leg (see figure 6.7a). Roll until you find a tender spot, and hold for about 30 seconds. When the time is up, roll through the muscle about four times.

Next, perform two motions, stretching the muscle by bending and extending the knee (see figure 6.7b). Repeat this process toward the top of the muscle in Zone 2.

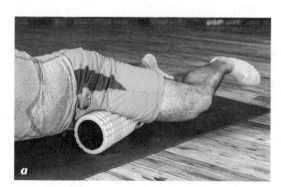
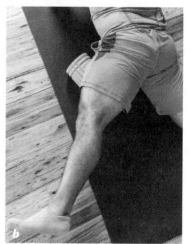

Figure 6.7 Adductors I: Roll up and down (a), and bend and extend (b).

ADDUCTORS EXERCISE II

This is an additional option for foam rolling the adductors. If you found considerable discomfort in Exercise I, then there is no need to perform this one. However, if you are experienced with foam rolling and are ready for a progression, then perform Adductors Exercise II. For this technique, use a slightly denser roller with a smaller diameter to influence more layers of tissue. Place the roller on top of a block to help elevate the roller into a more comfortable position.

Since this technique is a form of deep tissue foam rolling, it is important to divide the leg into three zones: Zone 1 will move from the knee to one-third of the way up the leg; Zone 2 will move from one-third to two-thirds of the way up the leg; and Zone 3 will move from two-thirds of the way up the leg to the hip.

Begin by lying face down. Place the foam roller next to you, with its long axis parallel to your body. Then, place the leg you are rolling over the roller. Place your forearms on the ground to support the upper body. To roll, slowly shift your body by lifting some pressure off of the floor and moving toward the roller so that the roller moves up the leg (see figure 6.8a). Roll until you find a tender spot, and hold for about 30 seconds. When the time is up, roll through the muscle about four times. Next, perform two motions, stretching the muscle by bending and extending the knee (see figure 6.8 b and c). Repeat this process near the middle of the muscle in Zone 2 and near the top of the muscle in Zone 3.

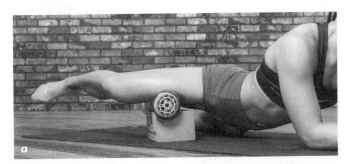

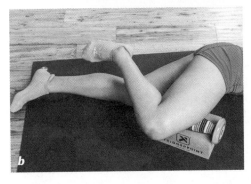
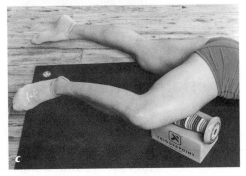

Figure 6.8 Adductors II: Roll up and down (a), and bend and extend (b and c).

IT BAND

The iliotibial (IT) band is an area of the body that seems to get significant attention. It is frequently the subject of many social media articles and always a hot debate at educational conferences and fitness events. It gets this attention because it is often wrongfully blamed for problems. The IT band does not start problems at all; rather, it tries to make up for muscles that fail on the job.

Basic Anatomy of the IT Band

The IT band is a band of connective tissue, like a ligament, that attaches to the hip bone (ilium), runs down the outside of the leg, and attaches to the tibia (see figure 6.9). Hence, the name including "ilio" and "tibial." Humans are not born with IT bands. Instead, humans begin with a layer of connective tissue called the fascia lata that surrounds the entire upper leg under the skin. At birth, the entire fascia lata has about the same thickness. Over time (and with our movement patterns such as crawling, walking, and running), the outside begins to thicken quicker than the rest of the tissue; this is the result of the tensor fasciae latae (TFL), a hip flexor muscle, and the gluteus maximus blending into this connective tissue. These are strong muscles that help with crawling, walking, and running. Thus, the more you move, the more force is transmitted down the leg and the thicker the connective tissue becomes. This is known as "Wolff's Law."

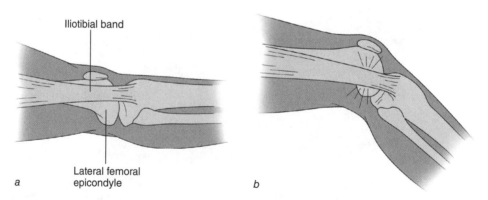

Figure 6.9 The IT band: extended knee *(a)* and bent knee *(b)*.

Function of the IT Band

The IT Band attaches to two important muscles: the gluteus maximus and the TFL (these will be discussed more in chapter 7). The IT band provides support and stabilization from the hips to the lower leg. When you walk or run, the hip muscles contract, creating tension in the IT band and transmitting the force down to the knee. This is why humans are able to run, with hundreds of pounds bearing down on one leg, yet still maintain a stable knee and pelvis. Essentially, the most important function of the IT band is stabilization. While ligaments, tendons, and other connective tissues, such as fascia, may have a very small ability to shorten, their shortening is a different process from that of the muscle. Muscles contract when they receive a signal from the nervous system. This helps you move from point A to point B along a path, in most cases. Other connective tissues cannot do this, as they lack the contractile components of a muscle. So, if there is a problem with the IT band, then you would need to address the muscles around it first.

Also, there is no such thing as a "tight" IT band, despite what you may have heard. Even if there was such a thing, it can't be stretched. The research on this is very clear. Humans are incapable of providing the force necessary to add any length to the IT band. Rumor suggests that two anatomists once used an IT band as a connection to pull a truck! Whether this is true, the point is that foam rolling or attempting to stretch the IT band will not add length to it.

Pros and Cons of Rolling the IT Band

If the IT band can't be stretched, then you may be thinking there's no point in using a foam roller on it. However, it is incredibly valuable—not because of the IT band but because of what lies beneath it. The largest and most powerful of the quadriceps (the vastus lateralis) lies directly under the IT band. To put it simply, when you think about rolling the IT band, know that you are really addressing the muscle under it. In fact, most of the pain you feel while rolling the IT band is rooted in the quadriceps. In addition, many times the vastus lateralis, being a large muscle, can compress into the IT band and give that sensation of tightness or pull on the outside of the knee. Again, rolling the IT band will decrease the tension in the vastus lateralis and relieve the pressure off the knee. This may give the illusion that you are releasing your IT band.

Foam Rolling Techniques for the IT Band

The preferred foam rolling technique for the IT band is very similar to that of the quadriceps, because essentially it is addressing one of the quadriceps. However, you will need to position yourself in a side plank to reach it. I recommend using a larger and softer roller to begin, due to the amount of pressure and the sensitivity of this area. This is not an area that many people feel needs additional pressure. Similar to quadriceps, divide the outside of the leg into two zones: Zone 1 involves rolling from the knee to halfway up the leg; Zone 2 involves rolling from halfway up the leg to the hip.

IT Band With Foam Roller

Begin by lying on your side on a smooth, comfortable surface. Next, place the leg over the roller so the outside of the upper leg is touching it. Position the roller just above the knee. Place your elbow and forearm just below the shoulder, and raise your hips up into a side plank. For extra stabilization, you can place the opposite arm and the leg you are not rolling out in front of you. If you desire extra pressure, stack your legs on top of each other. To begin rolling, move the body down so the roller moves up toward the hip at 1 inch, or 2.5 centimeters, per second (see figure 6.10a). If you find a tender spot, hold pressure for about 30 seconds. When the time is up, roll through the area about four times. Then, reposition the roller halfway up the leg, and stretch the muscle by bending and extending the knee about four times (see figure 6.10b). Repeat the process on the top half of the outside of the upper leg.

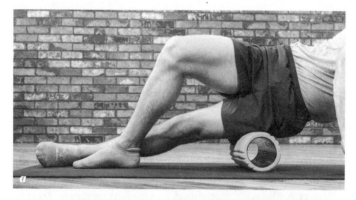

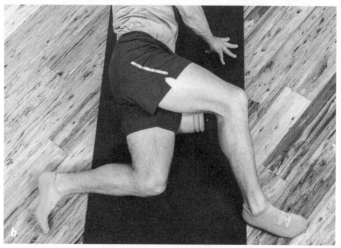

Figure 6.10 IT band: Roll up and down (a), and bend and extend (b).

Runner's Knee

Many people experience runner's knee, not just runners. The condition may be related to IT band problems or may be entirely unrelated. What the two have in common is pain. Whether you're dealing with a diagnosed condition of IT band syndrome or you have some general pain on the outside of the knee, I suggest you perform the same foam rolling techniques. If the knee hurts—anywhere on the knee—begin by foam rolling the quadriceps and adductors. Ideally, you should follow this with stretches and strengthening exercises. Not only can the quadriceps on the outside of the knee compress tissues and pull on the knee but also the quadriceps on the front can pull on the kneecap. This combination may cause the knee to experience jumper's knee, runner's knee, housemaid's knee, or any other type of painful knee condition.

The muscles of the upper leg are complex and powerful and can be problematic. If you follow a logical sequence and rationale to foam rolling these muscles, you can help relieve issues you didn't know were related. Of course, injury prevention and long-term high performance requires much more than just foam rolling the quadriceps. However, if everyone took just five minutes to focus on this area, it would likely play a significant role in decreasing injuries and pain.

Chapter 7

HIPS

For the purposes of this book, "hips" will be used to describe the muscles that are in close proximity to the pelvis. There are many muscles—45, according to Charles Thompson (2007), head athletic trainer at Princeton University — that attach to the pelvis. Therefore, this area has massive influence over how the rest of the body functions. Chapter 6 discussed many of the muscles that influence the hips, such as the quadriceps, hamstrings, and adductors.

The hips and the area around the pelvis have many sensitive spots. It is inadvisable to attempt to roll all muscles near the pelvis. This chapter will discuss the few that are easier to access and pose little risk when applying bodyweight compression: (1) the piriformis, which is beneath the gluteal complex on the posterior hip, (2) the gluteals, and (3) the tensor fascia latae muscle on the front of the hip. We will begin with the posterior aspect of the hip, the glutes and piriformis.

POSTERIOR HIP

For most people, foam rolling the hips is recommended. Whether due to working at a desk or the repetitive motions of a particular sport, the muscles are prone to problems. The body relies heavily on these muscles for stabilization and strength to walk, run, jump, and perform activities of daily living.

Basic Anatomy of the Posterior Hip

Several muscles compose the back of the hip, and the muscles in this area appear in layers (see figure 7.1). The deep muscles, which are hip rotators, are commonly called the "Deep Six" and are essentially three layers of gluteal muscles.

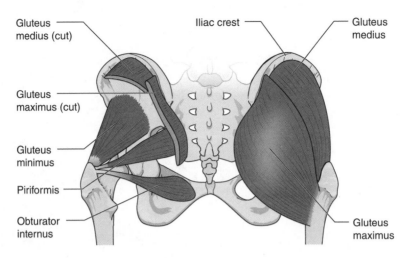

Gluteus medius (cut)

Iliac crest

Gluteus medius

Gluteus maximus (cut)

Gluteus minimus

Piriformis

Obturator internus

Gluteus maximus

Figure 7.1 Muscles of the posterior hip.

The muscles that make up the Deep Six are very similar to the rotator cuff of the shoulder. However, they do vary by function. All six of the hip rotators are external rotators, meaning when they shorten they can turn the knee outward. Of the six, the only muscle this book will discuss is the piriformis. The piriformis attaches to the front of the tailbone and runs almost completely horizontal to attach to the upper leg bone or femur. If this muscle worked in isolation, when it shortened, it would turn the leg out. This muscle may also assist in raising the leg out wide (abduction) and in extending the leg during walking. When this muscle is lengthening, it does the opposite: It resists internal rotation; hip flexion, to a degree; and hip adduction. It is important to understand that the length of the piriformis is related to the position of the knees and the pelvis.

In most people the knees cave inward when they squat or climb stairs or perform any activity on one leg. When the knees move inward, this lengthens the piriformis muscle along with most of the other posterior hip muscles. Muscles have a function much like a rubber band: The more you pull them, the tighter they become. Therefore, if the knees turn in, the piriformis is pulled long and feels tight. This may not initially sound like a big deal, but the body is designed to maintain normal posture and optimal alignment. If it is out of normal alignment, it will attempt to go back to normal. If the piriformis is long, it will want to shorten, so it will try to contract. The muscle is just doing its job—so what is wrong with that?

The sciatic nerve (discussed in chapter 3) happens to course through the piriformis and may get the raw end of the deal. This large nerve leaves the spine, runs through the hip muscles, in most cases runs directly through the piriformis, and provides sensation to the rest of the leg. If the piriformis contracts on the sciatic nerve, this can easily cause pain, numbness, and tingling down the leg. If you have any of these sensations, speak with a health care provider before foam rolling, as this may actually be caused by the spine itself. If you are cleared to foam roll, then it could provide massive relief.

The more recognizable muscle of the posterior hip, and the most powerful muscle in the body, is the gluteus maximus. In addition, it is the largest of any muscle, by mass and cross-sectional area. The gluteus maximus has many different attachments on the back of the body. It begins by attaching to the top of the pelvis and the sacrum and has fibers that are directed to the lateral side of the body on down. It also attaches to the leg, and a large part of the muscle attaches to the IT band. Additionally, the gluteus maximus has connective tissue that blends with the connective tissue of the latissimus dorsi muscle on the opposite side. This book won't go into extreme detail on this topic but know that the gluteus muscle on your right side helps to stabilize your left shoulder, and the gluteus muscle on your left side helps the right shoulder. All of these muscles and tissues work together to help stabilize areas of the low back.

As has been mentioned, it is important to make sure you're performing an assessment and rolling (and maybe stretching) muscles for a reason. The piriformis is one of those muscles that is often treated incorrectly. Foam rolling helps to reduce tension, which is great for a muscle that is pulled long. However, long muscles shouldn't be stretched—they are already long. The posterior hip is an area that is often stretched too much. Stretching a muscle that doesn't need additional length may temporarily decrease symptoms, but you must stretch every day to continue to find relief. Foam rolling and stretching should not be a "Band-Aid;" in other words, you shouldn't have to do it every day to keep pain at bay. If you must do it to function, you should probably explore the root cause of the problem.

Function of the Posterior Hip

For the most part, the muscles of the posterior hip have similar functions as what anatomy textbooks say. However, some of them have very distinct functions. Take, for example, the gluteus maximus.

The body of a professional sprinter seems close to ideal, in my opinion. Now, this may not be the perfect body to maintain in times of caloric hardship (muscle costs many calories), but it is close to ideal when it comes to human function. Humans are not the fastest animals, but we can reach our top speed quicker than most other animals. We are not the strongest (ants can lift more than 10 times their body weight), but we are strong for our size. We also don't have the most endurance compared to other species, but when trained correctly, humans can run up to 300 miles, or 482.8 kilometers, without stopping. Much of this can be attributed to the gluteus maximus and other large muscles such as the quadriceps. The gluteus maximus helps to extend the leg behind the body while also stabilizing the pelvis. In addition, the gluteus maximus is considered a "core" muscle due to its attachment to the pelvis and spine. This muscle should be large and powerful; unfortunately, it is commonly weak due to sedentary postures, dehydration, or simply a lack of understanding about the importance of training the gluteals.

In addition, there are also the Deep Six muscles under the gluteals, which serve as key external rotators of the hip. Their job is to first stabilize the leg in the hip joint and then to work to initiate external rotation as necessary. If the gluteus muscle is weak, then these muscles tend to do more. This may lead to compression of neural structures and other hip issues.

Pros and Cons of Rolling the Posterior Hip

Rolling the back of the hip can help you gain better function overall. Some muscles need to reduce tension (such as the piriformis); others need attention, hydration, and help with activation (as may be the case for the gluteus maximus). This chapter will help you focus on both of these as you roll. The first level will focus more on hydration, as putting pressure on the hip all day while sitting may force water and other fluids out of the area. Connective tissue specialist and researcher Robert Schleip suggests that by applying compression, stretching, and loading tissue the area can help you rehydrate better (Schleip et al., 2012). However, if the compression lasts for 12 to 14 hours per day, there will be no time for rehydration to occur. Therefore, some foam rolling and specific movements will help encourage fluids to move back into the area.

Foam Rolling Techniques for the Posterior Hip

To begin, slowly roll the area about 1 inch, or 2.5 centimeters, per second to identify any tender spots. A tender spot is something you identify as being painful or uncomfortable. As a general rule of thumb, on a scale of 1 (no pain) to 10 (worst pain imaginable), search for a spot that feels somewhere between a 5 and an 8. Less than a 5 may not be enough discomfort to encourage change, and any spots with pain greater than an 8 may involve too much pain to allow change. These tender spots may indicate that some type of adhesion, knot, or trigger point is present.

Once a spot is identified, relax the muscle that you are rolling and simply breathe into it. This should generally last for 30 to 60 seconds or until you feel a reduction in tenderness; then, add small motions. While each of these additional motions will differ depending on the body part you are rolling, most will follow the same pattern of trying to "pin and stretch" the muscle. You can do this by holding pressure and moving a joint close to the roller. Never roll up and down as quickly as possible.

Posterior Hip Exercise I

This technique uses a larger and slightly softer foam roller to cover more surface area and penetrate fewer layers of tissue. The area is divided into two zones: Zone 1 involves the more "meaty" area near the midway point of the glute; Zone 2 is higher, near the top of the hip, and works the superior fibers of the gluteus maximus. Muscles located deep beneath these areas will also be indirectly addressed because all tissue will be compressed.

Begin by placing the foam roller on a flat surface, and sit with one glute centered on the roller. Next, place at least one hand behind you for support while your feet are outstretched. Shift your weight to one side, with the body slightly rotated so more pressure is applied to one hip. Bend the leg you are not rolling so the foot is flat on the ground. The side that is being rolled can either be outstretched, or it can be crossed over the top of the other. I encourage you to try both positions to see which you prefer. Roll by slowly moving yourself downward so the roller moves up the glute at 1 inch, or 2.5 centimeters, per second (see figure 7.2a). If you find a tender spot, stop and hold for about 30 seconds. When the time is up, roll back through the muscle about four times; then, perform four to five hip flexion motions by raising the leg off the ground (see figure 7.2b).

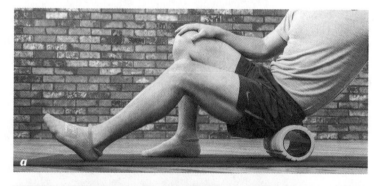

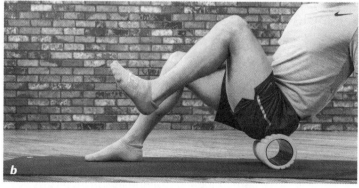

Figure 7.2 Posterior Hip I: Roll up and down (a), and flex the hip by raising the leg (b).

POSTERIOR HIP EXERCISE II

This technique uses a smaller and slightly harder roller to reach deeper and directly into the tissue. This technique more directly influences the piriformis than the previous technique. However, here it is important to apply compression, relax, and then work through the programming. Also, remember that the large sciatic nerve runs through the area. Applying compression to it is not dangerous, as long as it is not held for an extended amount of time. To be safe, I recommend that you spend no more than 60 to 90 seconds on each side.

Begin by placing a massage ball on a flat surface, and sit with one glute centered on the ball. Place your hands behind you for support, and bend the leg you are not rolling so the foot is flat on the floor, leaving the other leg outstretched. Shift your weight to one side, with the body slightly rotated so pressure is applied to one hip (see figure 7.3a). You will not roll as much here because, as you will see, the initial space where you place the ball is already tender. Breathe and relax into the massage ball for about 30 seconds or until the tenderness begins to decrease. When the time is up, perform four hip flexion motions by bringing the knee toward the chest (see figure 7.3b).

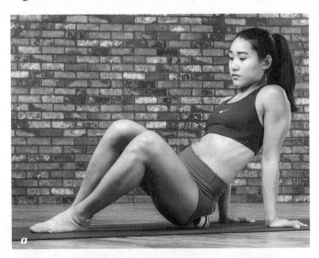

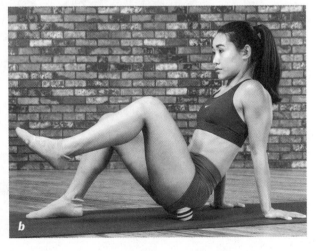

Figure 7.3 Posterior Hip II: Shift and apply pressure to the hip *(a)*, and flex the hip *(b)*.

ANTERIOR HIP

Foam rolling the back of the hip is a great way to start returning to optimal function. However, muscles on the front of the hip also frequently need attention. In many cases, the muscles on the front cause problems in the back.

Basic Anatomy of the Anterior Hip

As usual for the human body, many complex structures could play a role in dysfunction. However, they are challenging to access with a foam roller. So, the muscle to be most concerned about in the anterior hip—which is easy to access—is the tensor fascia latae, or TFL (see figure 7.4). The TFL is a small muscle in the front and side of the hip, with a long tendon that runs all the way down to the knee. This tendon is part of the IT band (discussed in chapter 6). As its name implies, the TFL increases tension in the fascia lata. The fascia lata is essentially the IT band and surrounding connective tissue of the upper leg. Thus, the TFL increases tension in the IT band, which then helps to stabilize both the pelvis and the knee.

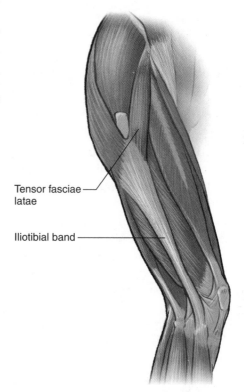

Tensor fasciae latae

Iliotibial band

Function of the Anterior Hip

The TFL attaches to the hip just behind a bony protrusion called the anterior superior iliac spine (ASIS). It then runs down a few inches and blends with the IT band. When the TFL contracts to shorten, it can flex the hip. Hip flexion occurs when the leg is raised in front of the body. If the foot is fixed firmly on the ground, the pelvis tilts anteriorly to flex

Figure 7.4 The TFL is a little muscle with major influence over hip mechanics.

the hip. This may contribute to low back pain if this position is maintained for long periods. Additionally, since the TFL attaches to the knee, it can internally rotate the upper leg and (oddly enough) externally rotate the lower leg. This is often a contributing factor in knee pain or injuries such as anterior cruciate ligament sprains and tears.

Pros and Cons of Rolling the Anterior Hip

As with all muscles, the muscles in the front of the hip adapt to do whatever they are asked to do most. In most people, these muscles are usually in a shortened position. When the TFL becomes adaptively shortened, it can pull the pelvis into an anterior pelvic tilt. The anterior pelvic tilt can put additional pressure on the low back and play a large part in chronic low back pain. Therefore, in most of the population, it is important to release this muscle.

Additionally, because of the attachments of this muscle, it may put extra pressure on the knee. When the TFL is short and tight, it tenses the IT band and increases the compression to parts of the knee. The current leading theory to explain runner's knee and IT band syndrome points to excessive compression on the highly innervated fat pad on the outside of the knee. Again, spending a few minutes on the TFL before a workout or even simply after a long day at the office may help to reduce the chance of injury and increase performance.

Foam Rolling Techniques for the Anterior Hip

To begin, slowly roll the area about 1 inch, or 2.5 centimeters, per second to identify any tender spots. The muscles of the anterior hip are not as large as the others, so there will be very small rolling motions performed. A tender spot is something you identify as being painful or uncomfortable. As a general rule of thumb, on a scale of 1 (no pain) to 10 (worst pain imaginable), search for a spot that feels somewhere between a 5 and an 8. Less than a 5 may not be enough discomfort to encourage change, and any spots with pain greater than an 8 may involve too much pain to allow change. These tender spots may indicate that some type of adhesion, knot, or trigger point is present.

Once you identify a spot, relax the muscle that is being rolled and simply breathe into it. This should generally last for 30 to 60 seconds or until you feel a reduction in tenderness; then, add some small motions. While each of these additional motions will be different depending on the body part you are rolling, most will follow the same pattern of trying to "pin and stretch" the muscle. You can do this by holding pressure and moving a joint close to the roller. Never roll up and down as quickly as possible.

ANTERIOR HIP EXERCISE I

This technique uses a regular-sized foam roller. Begin by locating the muscle, remembering that the muscle is just below the crest of the hip. Place the foam roller on a flat surface, and lie down with the roller directly on the muscle. If this muscle is problematic, there is a good chance that just lying there will be uncomfortable; there may not be a need to roll in an attempt to find a tender spot. A regular foam roller will apply pressure directly to the TFL. If it is not initially tender, try to reposition yourself by moving the hips in and out or by slowly rolling the muscle about one 1, or 2.5 centimeters, per second. Once you find a tender spot, hold pressure for about 30 seconds. When the time is up, add a little movement by performing hip rotations. First, bend the knee to about 90 degrees, then allow the foot to fall out toward the ground; this will internally rotate the hip (see figure 7.5a). Then, bring the foot back up to externally rotate the hip (see figure 7.5b). Perform this four to five times.

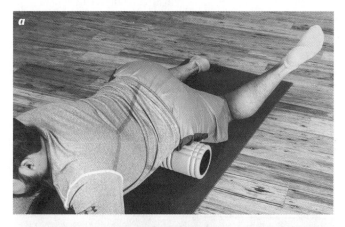

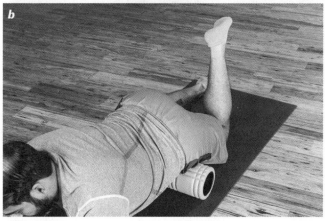

Figure 7.5 Anterior Hip I: Internally rotate the hip *(a)*, and externally rotate the hip *(b)*.

ANTERIOR HIP EXERCISE II

This technique uses a massage ball that is 5 inches, or 12.7 centimeters, in diameter; is harder than a foam roller; and has less surface area so it gets deeper, influencing more layers of tissue. Only move on to this technique if you have been working on Anterior Hip Exercise I for several weeks. As with Exercise I, the TFL is likely going to be uncomfortable as soon as you apply pressure.

Begin by placing a massage ball on a flat surface. Then lie on the ball so the center of the TFL is directly on the ball. Similar to Exercise I, this initial position is probably going to be the tender spot. If so, relax and breathe, holding pressure for about 30 seconds or until the tenderness begins to decrease. If it is not tender, then search the area by rolling up, down, or side to side at 1 inch, or 2.5 centimeters, per second. Once a tender spot is found, hold still. After the time is up, add a little movement by performing hip rotations. First, bend the knee to about 90 degrees, then allow the foot to fall out toward the ground; this will internally rotate the hip (see figure 7.6a). Then, bring the foot back up to externally rotate the hip (see figure 7.6b). Perform this four to five times.

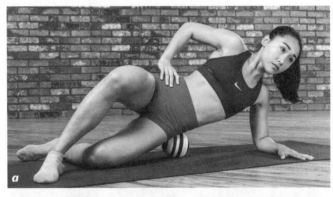

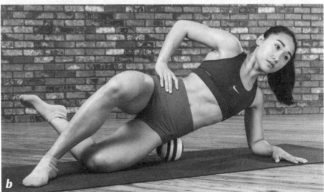

Figure 7.6 Anterior Hip II: Internally rotate the hip (a), and externally rotate hip (b).

The muscles around the hip have a large influence over the rest of the body. They work to produce power for walking, running, and jumping. They also work to stabilize the core. In addition, these muscles must function optimally to ensure proper stabilization of the feet and even the shoulders. Spending even a few minutes on these muscles several times a week will likely help you to feel and move better.

Chapter 8

CHEST AND UPPER BACK

The chest and back are areas that you may not think of as tight or dysfunctional, especially the chest. While it is not uncommon for the upper back (and neck) to express feelings of tightness, the muscles of the upper back are rarely responsible for any trouble. Usually the muscles on the front, the chest muscles, need the foam rolling and stretching, while the muscles on the back usually need to be strengthened. It can be a little tricky to determine where to roll the upper back. This chapter will briefly describe these areas, explore why you may or may not need to roll them, and help address each area with a foam roller for the best results.

CHEST

The muscles of the chest can create many problems in someone who performs repetitive movements or has bad posture. As you will soon see, most of these muscles do plenty of work through daily activity, and they likely only need special attention when they get tight.

Basic Anatomy of the Chest

There are four specific muscles that make up the chest, two on each side. These muscles, collectively known as the pectorals, attach to the ribs, shoulders, and arms. The pectorals are found on the front of the body toward the top of the rib cage. Consider, first, the pectoralis major.

The pectoralis major is the larger of the two muscles on each side. It begins (or originates) at the ribs, sternum, and clavicle; it ends (or inserts) onto the upper arm bone. As such, this muscle can create movement around all these

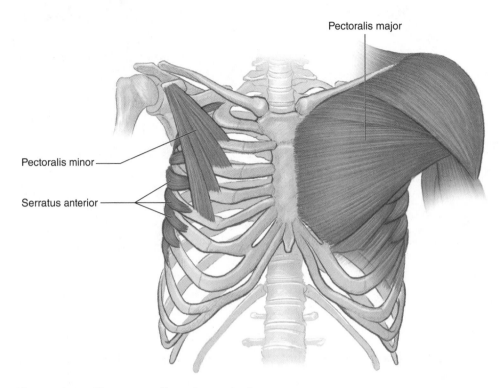

Figure 8.1 The pectoralis major and minor.

joints. Under the pectoralis major is the smaller pectoralis minor. It lies under the larger muscle, attaching again to the ribs but then also attaching to the shoulder blade. This muscle has a key influence on the ribs and the shoulder blade, but only has an indirect influence on the movement of the arm. Figure 8.1 illustrates the pectoralis major and pectoralis minor.

Function of the Chest

The muscles of the chest, pectoralis major and pectoralis minor, work together to coordinate and control the movement of the arm. The pectoralis major, which actually attaches to the arm, will work to bring the arm toward the front of the body, inwardly rotate the arm, and (if the arm is high enough) bring the arm back down. Since this muscle attaches to the ribs, it may assist with rib motion. Of course, the motion in the ribs is less than in the arm; but, if the arm is fixed, as it is when you hang from a pull-up bar, then it will bring the ribs closer to the arm. Additionally, the muscles of the pectoralis major can work when the arm is really far behind you. Imagine reaching to the back seat of a car. When the body is rotated and one arm is reaching backward, it puts a significant stretch on these muscles.

The pectoralis minor has a much different function. This muscle does not actually attach to the arm but to the shoulder blade. Therefore, its influence on the arm is only indirect, as it moves the shoulder blade. However, that doesn't mean it's not important—it may be a more important factor in problems than the pectoralis major. Anatomy textbooks often mention that the pectoralis minor depresses the shoulder blade, as well as protracts and elevates the ribs. Protraction is the movement of the shoulder blades away from the spine. If you were seated and needed to reach for something far in front of you, so far that you would need to stretch to grasp it, your shoulder would need to protract. However, in the real world, the pectoralis minor alone does little to contribute to this.

The pectoralis minor does protract but only with the help of another very important muscle—the serratus anterior. You can think of this muscle as the opposite of the pectoralis minor but also its coworker. Together, they pull the shoulder blade around the rib cage and toward the front. However, this relationship is often a rocky one. In many cases the pectoralis begins doing much more than it should. This upsets the serratus, which begins doing less than its fair share. The result is not protraction but an anterior tipping of the shoulder blade. Anterior tipping happens when the top of the shoulder blade moves forward, and the bottom of the shoulder blade moves backward. The easiest way to tell if you have this condition is to look at yourself from the side, in a mirror. You will need to have a view of your shoulder blade, so it is necessary to wear a tank top or take your shirt off. From this side angle, your shoulder blade should appear flat. An anteriorly tipped shoulder blade will be rotated forward. If you see the bottom of the shoulder blade (inferior angle) poking out, off the rib cage, this is a common sign of anterior tipping. Of course, anterior tipping is normal for certain motions, such as extending your arms behind you as far as you can; but if the shoulder blade is always in this position, it may lead to shoulder impingement.

It is always important to be aware of nerves and other important structures. Similar to the relationship between the sciatic nerve and the piriformis, there is a bundle of nerves near the pectoralis minor: the brachial plexus. The brachial plexus houses all the nerves that innervate the arm. Thus, if the pectoralis minor is dysfunctional, there is a small chance it may compress the nerves. If you are having arm or shoulder pain, don't just begin rolling those areas. Speak with an educated trainer, therapist, or your physician first.

Pros and Cons of Rolling the Chest

If the pectoralis minor is dysfunctional—disturbing normal function of the serratus anterior and causing anterior tipping of the scapula—it sets the stage for shoulder impingement. You might say that the root cause of this spiraling dysfunction is a faulty diaphragm, which is correct. However, it is inadvisable to perform self-diaphragm release (see a manual therapist for this). It is safe, on the other hand, to perform pectoralis minor release.

The pectoralis major is not as dysfunctional as the pectoralis minor appears to be. However, this muscle can be problematic in someone with rounded forward posture. As previously mentioned, the pectoralis major is a primary

INTRODUCTION TO BREATHING

The pectoralis minor is considered a secondary respiratory muscle. During forced inhalation, such as while running sprints up and down a hill, the pectoral muscle contracts to lift the ribs, allowing the lungs to expand upward. Please note that this is a *secondary* respiratory muscle. While detailed breathing function is beyond the scope of this book, it should be mentioned briefly here. After all, breathing is kind of a big deal.

The diaphragm is one of the most important muscles in breathing (see figure 8.2). The diaphragm attaches to the bottom of the ribs, parts of the spine, and the bottom of the lungs. When this muscle contracts, it pulls the lungs down, allowing for proper expansion during inhalation. When breathing is very rapid (as it might be while running sprints), then the body calls on additional muscles to assist (such as the pectoralis minor). This is considered normal. However, when these additional muscles are called into action and you are not performing higher intensity activity, then it is considered dysfunctional. This is often referred to as apical breathing and can be caused by poor posture, excessive stress, or improper breathing techniques learned over time.

People who don't know how to properly breathe may be in a chronic state of breathing dysfunction. Often, the diaphragm becomes stuck, unable to properly contract or relax. When the diaphragm doesn't do its job, the body always reverts back to a secondary method—especially for something as important as breathing. In this case, the pectoralis minor (secondary respiratory muscle) works harder and lifts the rib cage more. After approximately 20,000 breaths a day, the pectoralis minor becomes overworked, hypertrophic, and unable to extend to its normal length.

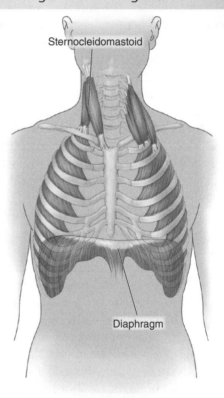

Figure 8.2 The diaphragm and its attachment to the ribs and spine.

internal rotator of the arm. Internal rotation happens, for example, when you begin with your palm facing forward, then rotate it inward so it faces your thigh, and then continue rotating so the palm faces behind you. If you were to rotate inward day-in and day-out, then the pectoralis major can entangle itself with many of the other muscles in the area, such as the deltoids or biceps. Many connective tissue problems occur in this area. In addition, the pectoralis major is notorious for having trigger points and knots that form closer to the sternum. However, this book will focus more on rolling toward the tip of the shoulder, offering extra attention to the pectoralis minor and the collection of connective tissue.

Foam Rolling Techniques for the Chest

Foam rolling the muscles in the chest involves a slightly different program than the other areas of the body. Since the target area is relatively small, you will not need to do as much actual rolling. Instead, pressure will be applied directly to the center of the muscle. While you are more than welcome to search around, in most cases where the pressure is applied first is the most tender.

Once a spot is identified, relax the muscle that is being rolled and breathe into it. This should generally last for 30 to 60 seconds or until you feel a reduction in tenderness; then, add small motions. To address the pectoralis minor, I have found that simple arm sweeps are the easiest and most valuable motions to perform. If, while rolling or holding pressure, you begin to feel numbness or tingling in the arm or hand, you may be compressing the nerves. Don't be alarmed, but you should change your position to take the pressure off the nerve.

CHEST WITH FOAM ROLLER

Begin rolling the chest with a normal-sized foam roller. The recommended position will allow you to target both the pectoralis major and minor; with a larger size roller, more emphasis will be placed on the pectoralis major. Lay the foam roller on a flat surface and lie face down next to it. Place the roller at about a 45-degree angle near the tip of the shoulder. Apply more pressure onto the roller by shifting your body weight onto it. This position is safe for both men and women. As stated previously, you will not be making large rolling motions with these muscles. Therefore, you will not be compressing excessive amounts of breast tissue, as you are essentially just to the outside of it. If the area is tender, relax into it for about 30 seconds. If you need to search for a tender spot, use your opposite arm to slowly move you across the roller at about 1 inch, or 2.5 centimeters, per second until you find a spot, and then hold. When the time is up, perform four small rolling motions side to side (see figure 8.3a). This often involves a simple rocking motion. Next, perform four to five arm sweeps by lifting the arm off the ground and moving it from near your head to down toward your side (see figure 8.3b). Maintain pressure on the roller the entire time.

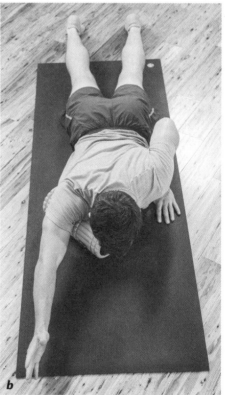

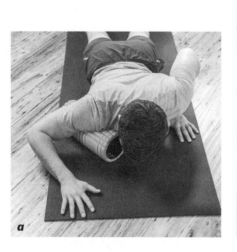

Figure 8.3 Chest with foam roller: Roll side to side *(a)*, and sweep the arm *(b)*.

CHEST WITH MASSAGE BALL

Using a large massage ball to roll the chest involves a similar experience to rolling with a regular foam roller. However, the ball puts more direct pressure on the body, so only advance to this technique when you feel you are ready. This technique targets the pectoralis minor under the pectoralis major.

Begin by laying the ball on a flat surface, and then lie face down. Place the ball under the chest, toward the tip of the shoulder. Note that the ball should not be on the tip of the shoulder but just to the inside and slightly below, directly on the intended muscle. Apply more pressure if needed by rotating your body into the massage ball while keeping the arm relaxed. If you feel a tender spot, hold for about 30 seconds. If you need to roll the area to find a tender spot, use the opposite arm to perform small rolling motions. Once the time is up, roll through the area four times. Do this by using the opposite arm to shift the body side to side (see figure 8.4a). Then, perform four to five arm sweeps by lifting the hand off the ground and bringing it down toward your side and back up (see figure 8.4b).

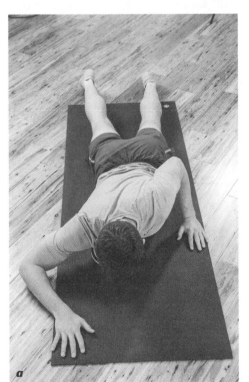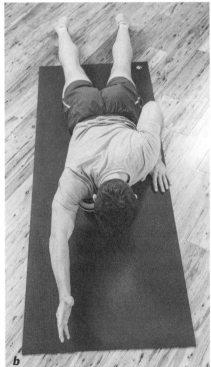

Figure 8.4 Chest with massage ball: Roll side to side (a), and sweep the arm (b).

UPPER BACK

The upper back feels great during rolling. Foam rolling can help reduce tension and stress, aid breathing, and is especially valuable to those who work in a seated position all day. In a way, you can think of the muscles in this area like the hamstrings, because they are often pulled tight. Instead of trying to stretch these muscles, you may need to increase blood flow and perhaps strengthen them.

Basic Anatomy of the Back

When discussing the back, this chapter will refer specifically to the upper back. The lower back, as mentioned earlier in the book, should be left to the professionals. The upper back is covered with several layers of muscles. The thoracic spine makes up the middle segment of the vertebral column (see figure 8.5). It lies between the cervical spine (neck) and the lumbar spine (low back). There are 12 vertebrae in the thoracic spine. Posture, stress, poor breathing, and a lack of movement can cause this area to become stuck and tight. In order to move and function properly, each portion of the spine needs to be able to move the way it was designed. Therefore, the thoracic spine needs to be able to rotate to properly transmit forces through the body.

The muscles that cover the upper back, beginning with the deeper muscles, are the rhomboids and the trapezius. The rhomboids attach to the spine and then extend outward to the shoulder blade (see figure 8.6). They are not the deepest of the upper back muscles, but they are the deepest muscles that a foam roller can influence. Under the rhomboids are very small muscles that generally serve to attach one vertebrae to another. These are too small to be foam rolled. In most anatomy textbooks, the rhomboids are divided into two separate muscles: The smaller muscle is the rhomboid minor, and the larger is the rhomboid major. However, for foam rolling purposes, this book will consider them as one muscle.

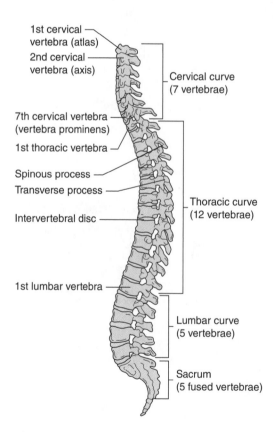

1st cervical vertebra (atlas)
2nd cervical vertebra (axis)
Cervical curve (7 vertebrae)
7th cervical vertebra (vertebra prominens)
1st thoracic vertebra
Spinous process
Transverse process
Intervertebral disc
Thoracic curve (12 vertebrae)
1st lumbar vertebra
Lumbar curve (5 vertebrae)
Sacrum (5 fused vertebrae)

Figure 8.5 The thoracic spine.

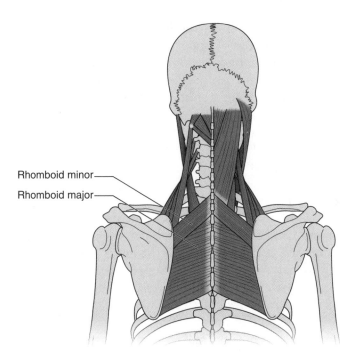

Figure 8.6 The rhomboids.

The trapezius muscle lies across the top of the rhomboids (see figure 8.7). Commonly referred to as the "traps," this one large muscle is shaped like a trapezoid. While it is one muscle, it has many different muscle fibers that run in different directions; therefore, it is usually described as the lower trap, middle trap, and upper trap. The trapezius attaches to the base of the skull, runs down the spine to the bottom of the thoracic spine (bottom of the rib cage), and then extends outward to attach to the entire top of the shoulder blade.

Function of the Upper Back

The upper back is an area of the spine designed for rotation. This rotation is vital for proper function of the shoulder and arm, stabilization of the head and

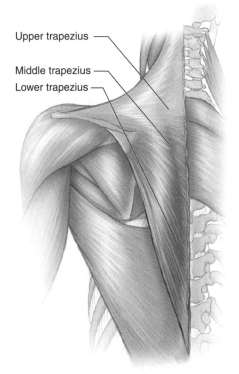

Figure 8.7 The trapezius.

neck, and transfer of forces from the lower body through the upper body. Extension is another function of upper back motion that frequently becomes dysfunctional. Our spine is made to move in all directions, albeit some directions are easier than others. In our sedentary and sometimes stressful world, many people slouch. Slouching is spinal flexion. If we are slouched too often, then we begin to lose the ability to extend. Upper back extension is vital to ideal arm movement. If you'd like to feel this movement, try to slowly reach both arms over your head. As you do this, pay attention to the motion the upper back is going through. You will notice that it must extend for both arms to get overhead.

The rhomboids and the trapezius muscles work together, primarily to stabilize the shoulder blade but also to assist in movement. When you reach overhead, the rhomboids and trapezius muscles stabilize the shoulder blade and assist in guiding it along the correct path until the arms are up. Many people with shoulder impingement have lost this coordinated, upward rotation. It's important to note that these muscles are rarely short and tight. In most people, they are pulled long and weak or are underactive. If we consider that common forward, rounded posture, the shoulder blades are usually rotated forward. This position lengthens these muscles. This may make rhomboids and trapezius muscles feel tight, but as we have learned, muscles that feel tight are rarely short and tight.

Pros and Cons of Rolling the Upper Back

Introducing, or reintroducing, motion back into this area is key to restoring function to the entire spine. You will roll the rhomboids and trapezius muscles—but the goal is not necessarily to release these muscles. As you roll, you will be bringing fresh blood and oxygen to the muscles, but the focus will be on reintroducing that ideal extension and rotation to the upper back. Then, you can target these long and usually weak muscles with a strengthening program. As the National Academy of Sports Medicine suggests, for a corrective exercise routine for the back and shoulder, if you strengthen the muscles of the upper back, it will lead to better shoulder stabilization and function (Clark & Lucett, 2011).

Chapter 9, which covers the shoulders, will discuss one of the largest muscles in the back that is usually short and problematic. In fact, most of the muscles that lead to upper back tightness and discomfort attach to the shoulder. These muscles that feel tight are usually lengthened. While you can foam roll these, rolling them doesn't usually fix anything. Therefore, to really relieve the upper back, you should target this area of the spine by performing a thoracic spine movement technique.

Foam Rolling Techniques for the Upper Back

Foam rolling the upper back does not usually lead to the same discomfort as you might experience with other areas of the body. This can be explained by the fact that these muscles aren't usually short and tight but are long and dysfunctional. Rolling this area feels great!

UPPER BACK EXERCISE I

This technique uses a regular-sized foam roller. Since this type of roller covers more surface area, you can roll the upper back as one zone. Begin by placing the foam roller on a flat surface. Sit next to it and lie back so the roller is positioned at the bottom of the shoulder blades. This exercise will target from the bottom of the shoulder blades to the top of the shoulder blades. Take caution not to roll down into the lower back or up onto the neck. Position your arms behind your head for support. It is important to try to relax the muscles on the front of the body to get the most benefit. Bend the hips and knees so the feet are flat on the ground. Next, position your upper back into a slight extension by allowing the shoulder, head, and neck to lower over the roller a small amount. I suggest your face and chest be pointed directly toward the ceiling.

To begin rolling, raise your hips off the ground a bit; then, pull yourself down with your legs so the foam roller moves up the back at 1 inch, or 2.5 centimeters, per second (see figure 8.8a). You may not feel much tenderness, but if you do, hold pressure for about 30 seconds. It is common to hear some popping or cracking in this area as the ribs may adjust when you roll across. Roll through the areas slowly about four times. Next, roll yourself to position the roller about midway up the shoulder blades, and set your hips on the ground. Perform four to five cross-friction motions, sliding the upper back side to side across the roller (see figure 8.8b). To do this, imagine you are trying to touch your right elbow to your right knee, and then the left elbow to the left knee. This will create a sliding motion across the foam roller. A word of caution here: Many people who are just beginning will roll very aggressively and end up with red marks or small bruises on the upper back. If this happens, reduce the amount of pressure on the roller by keeping the hips on the ground while rolling.

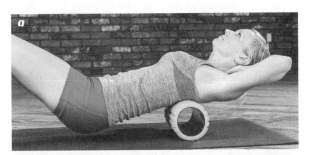

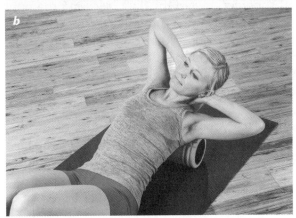

Figure 8.8 Upper back I: Roll up the back (a), and slide side to side (b).

UPPER BACK EXERCISE II

For this technique, I suggest dividing the upper back into three zones: Zone 1 involves rolling near the bottom of the shoulder blades; Zone 2 involves rolling near the middle of the shoulder blades; and Zone 3 involves rolling near the top of the shoulder blades. Each zone area is about 1 to 1.5 inches, or 2.5 to 3.8 centimeters. You will roll up and down on the massage balls, so two techniques will be performed in each zone.

To begin, place two massage balls next to each other on a flat surface. Many people like to place the massage balls in a sleeve or sock (commonly referred to as a "peanut") to keep them together. Sit in front of the massage balls and lie back so one ball is on each side of the spine. First, target Zone 1 near the bottom of the shoulder blades. Once in position, try to lie your head and shoulders back so they are relaxed on the ground. This position can often be uncomfortable; so if you need, grab a yoga block or a regular foam roller to use as a pillow the first few times. Similar to Upper Back Exercise I, you will need to relax the muscles on the front of the body so you can move the spine. If you are activating all of these muscles by holding the head and shoulders up, then you are reducing the effectiveness of the technique. Bend the hips and knees so the feet are on the floor. This will help relax the lower back and take tension off of the hip flexors.

You will not roll here, so there is no need to search for a tender spot and hold it. Instead, take a few seconds here to breathe and relax into the massage balls. Next, perform four to five rotations. Do this by crossing your hands in front of your chest and placing them lightly on the shoulders. Then, while keeping your hips stationary, rotate the shoulders (see figure 8.9a). This should be a small motion, but try to move the right shoulder back toward the floor as the left shoulder comes up off the floor. Then repeat on the other side by moving the left shoulder toward the floor, allowing the right shoulder to come up. Move slowly and breathe through each motion. After completing these shoulder rotations, perform four to five shoulder flexion motions (see figure 8.9b). Do this by reaching both hands toward the sky; then slowly reach for the ground over your head. The goal is not to touch the ground but to get as close as you can. Then, bring the arms back out in front. Repeat this four to five times.

Next, reposition to Zone 2. Place your arms beside you for assistance, raising your hips and using your legs to pull you down so the massage balls move up 1 to 2 inches, or 2.5 or 5 centimeters. Move slowly. Then, repeat the rotation and shoulder flexion. Lastly, move to Zone 3, and repeat the motions.

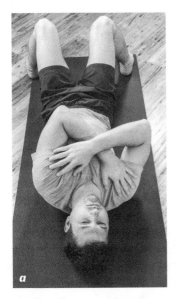 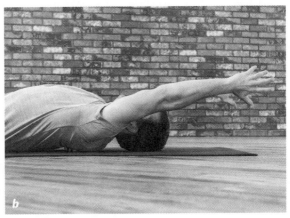

Figure 8.9 Upper back II: Rotate the shoulder *(a)*, and flex the shoulder *(b)*.

If you are frustrated that this book does not cover foam rolling for all muscles of the back, remember that you do not need to roll every muscle. I recommend you refrain from always targeting muscles that feel tight, as these sensations are often misleading. If you are feeling that common upper back and neck discomfort, the two techniques described in this chapter will help a great deal. However, to truly relieve that tension, you should move on to the techniques discussed in chapter 9.

Chapter 9

SHOULDERS AND ARMS

Chapter 8 covered some important areas that contribute to the majority of the aches and pains in the neck and shoulders. However, there are additional muscles that play a role in optimal shoulder and arm function. If you have any shoulder or arm pain, I suggest you begin with the techniques described in chapter 8. Once you've completed those movements, then you can move on to the techniques described in this chapter.

This chapter covers some often-forgotten muscles that frequently contribute to common aches and pains. The shoulder is one of the most complex joints in the body. In normal human movement patterns, the shoulder begins as a joint needed for stability. For example, by about 3 months old, a child begins to prop itself up on their elbows and quickly after begins to crawl. Thus, the shoulder joint is demonstrating stability. However, soon after that, the child begins to stand, walk, and run. Now, the shoulder is no longer being used for stability and is able to fulfill its more primary role for mobility. Therefore, the more than 20 muscles that directly affect shoulder function have a lot of work to do. A few of these muscles, namely the biceps, aren't usually considered as a part of the shoulders. However, the biceps cross the shoulder joint and therefore affect the shoulder.

This chapter will also cover the muscles of the forearm. In my opinion, both the flexors and extenders pick up a lot of slack for other muscles. They generally work overtime with a faulty shoulder to attempt to offer the most normal movement possible at the wrist and hand. After placing the shoulder, elbow, and wrist in a less than optimal position for many hours, days, or even years, the forearm muscles will need attention.

SHOULDER

The shoulder is a simple ball-and-socket joint, yet it has a complex overall function and the body often demands a lot from it. The shoulder is one of the most injured body parts and, interestingly, there is rarely ever direct contact or trauma to it. That means that much of the shoulder pain plaguing our society may be avoidable. The first step to optimal function is to understand the basic function and anatomy of the shoulder.

Basic Anatomy of the Shoulder

As explained in chapter 8, the thoracic spine is an integral part of shoulder anatomy. To reiterate, if the upper back cannot move properly, then the shoulder blade and entire shoulder will also be dysfunctional. Many cases of shoulder impingement, which is the most common disorder of the shoulder (Silva et al., 2008), are linked to thoracic spine problems. The shoulder blade interacts with the ribs and the ribs interact with the spine.

The shoulder is not one specific bone or joint but an area of the body. The upper quarter and top of the arm house a complex interaction of many bones and muscles, which make up the shoulder girdle. More specifically, the shoulder girdle comprises of the scapula (shoulder blade) and the clavicle. The clavicle is a small bone that connects the shoulder blade to the sternum, which is near the rib cage. Incredibly, this little bone serves as the only "hard" attachment site for the entire upper arm. Apart from that, we rely on the coordination of about 17 different muscles to keep our arm in place. Because of this, shoulder injuries and nagging pain are common in our society. It is likely that if we used our shoulders for much more, as intended, like crawling and climbing for example, the rates of shoulder pain would be much less.

When most people think of the shoulder joint, they think solely of the glenohumeral joint (see figure 9.1). This is the joint where the upper arm bone (humerus) attaches to the shoulder blade (glenoid fossa). The glenohumeral joint is the most mobile joint in the entire body. However, other joints also reside in the shoulder. The body also has the joints created by the clavicle and the shoulder blade (acromioclavicular, or AC, joint), the joint created by the clavicle and the sternum (sternoclavicular joint), and the joint created by the scapula on the rib cage (scapulothoracic joint). While most people rarely think of these joints, they are equally important in the function of the shoulder. If one of these joints does not

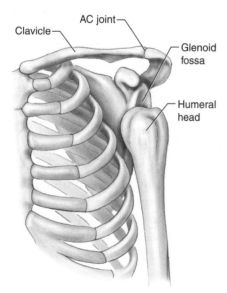

Clavicle

AC joint

Glenoid fossa

Humeral head

Figure 9.1 The shoulder girdle.

move optimally, the others will have to compensate. This compensation can lead to aches, pains, and injury.

Of course, the bones and joints alone do not typically cause problems. It is the muscles that attach to these bones that are overactive (tight) or underactive (weak) and pull the everything out of alignment. These muscles include the pectoralis minor (already discussed in chapter 8) and the serratus anterior (see figure 9.2a), the posterior deltoid (see figure 9.2b), the trapezius and latissimus dorsi (see figure 9.2c), and the levator scapulae and rhomboids (see figure 9.2d).

The latissimus dorsi is one of the largest muscles in the body. It is not necessarily thick, like the gluteus maximus, but it is wide. This muscle begins on the back of the pelvis and runs upward, attaching to the lower back, the bottom few ribs, a small piece of the shoulder blade, and (at its end) the front of the upper arm bone. Any muscle covering this much surface area and crossing this many joints is likely to experience some problems over time. The latissimus dorsi often contributes not only to shoulder problem, but also low back problems.

Next is the levator scapulae, a little muscle that attaches to the top of the shoulder blade and runs upward toward the base of the skull. As the name implies, when this muscle shortens, it elevates the scapula. However, if the scapula doesn't elevate, for whatever reason, then this muscle will tug on the neck and head. When someone complains of "knots in the neck," this is usually the prime suspect. However, this muscle does not usually cause the problem. It is generally just adapting to the position the body is in most of the time.

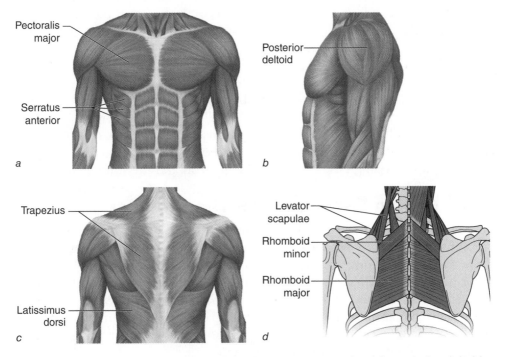

Figure 9.2 Muscles of the shoulder girdle: serratus anterior *(a)*, posterior deltoid *(b)*, trapezius and latissimus dorsi *(c)*, and levator scapulae and rhomboids *(d)*.

The last muscle to discuss here is the posterior deltoid. This muscle is found on the back of the shoulder. The literal interpretation of posterior deltoid is "the back of the triangle" because the three muscles that make up the deltoids form an upside-down triangle. This muscle is tricky like the hamstrings. When someone has forward posture, for example, this muscle is usually pulled and lengthened.

Function of the Shoulder

The shoulder is strategically designed to handle a variety of motions. The shoulder joint where the upper arm and scapula meet (glenohumeral joint) can move in all directions. Considering only forward and backward movement, a healthy joint is capable of more than 240 degrees of total motion. It's called a "ball-and-socket" joint because it looks as though a ball would fit into the socket. However, the shoulder joint is designed more like a golf ball sitting on a tee. The way the socket is designed does not allow the top of the arm to fit securely. While this allows the body to enjoy movement, it can also allow shoulder impingement. The most common form of shoulder pain is caused by the arm bone sliding forward and pressing on other muscles, nerves, and tissues in the joint. Over time, the tissues become irritated, inflamed, and painful.

Pros and Cons of Rolling the Shoulder

It should be apparent now that most people will need to roll the shoulder. People don't always use the shoulder for what it was made for, and repetitive postures cause the muscles around the shoulder to become short and problematic. To begin with, the latissimus dorsi will, if you are slouching, become short and pull the upper arm into an inwardly rotated position. If left for too long, this position may compress many of the tissues in this region. This position also pulls the back of the shoulder into a stretched position and lengthens the posterior deltoid. In an effort to try to stabilize the shoulder, it still contracts and becomes chronically engaged. You do not need to stretch this muscle; rather, you can foam roll it and move on. The last muscle that needs attention here is the levator scapulae. When the body is slouched forward, this muscle contracts in an attempt to realign the eyes with the horizon and the stabilize the head.

Foam Rolling Techniques for the Shoulder

To begin, slowly roll the shoulder at about 1 inch, or 2.5 centimeters, per second to identify any tender spots. A tender spot is something you identify as being painful or uncomfortable. As a general rule of thumb, on a scale of 1 (no pain) to 10 (worst pain imaginable), search for a spot that feels somewhere between a 5 and an 8. Less than a 5 may not be enough discomfort to encourage change, and any spots with pain greater than an 8 may involve too much pain to allow change. These tender spots may indicate that some type of adhesion, knot, or trigger point is present.

Once a spot is identified, relax the muscle that is being rolled and simply breathe into it. This should generally last for 30 to 60 seconds or until you feel a reduction in tenderness; then, add small motions. While each of these additional motions will be different depending on the body part you are rolling, most will follow the same pattern of trying to "pin and stretch" the muscle. This happens by holding pressure and moving a joint close to the roller. Never roll up and down as quickly as possible.

LATISSIMUS DORSI WITH FOAM ROLLER

The latissimus dorsi covers the majority of the back. However, most of the back is somewhat sensitive. Therefore, it is best to target the area near the arm.

To begin, lie on your side on a flat, comfortable surface. Stack the legs, and add a slight bend so the hips and knees are relaxed. Then, place the foam roller under the latissimus dorsi, which is about midway up the rib cage, while still sharing some pressure with the shoulder blade. Begin rolling up and down until you find a tender spot and hold (see figure 9.3a). While holding, perform the arm sweep by reaching the arm directly in front of your body. I typically recommend rotating the shoulder so the palm is facing upward, as this is often more comfortable. Next, keep the muscle pinned and sweep the arm upward, toward your head, until the shoulder is fully flexed (see figure 9.3b). If there is any pain in the shoulder joint while sweeping, then you don't have to go all the way. Only move the shoulder as far as is comfortable, realizing there may naturally be some discomfort from the foam roller.

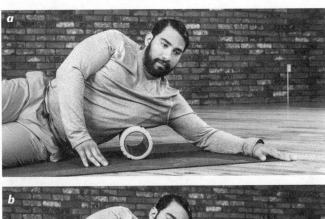

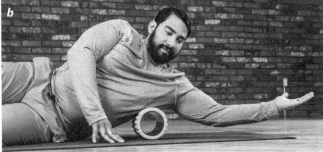

Figure 9.3 Latissimus dorsi with foam roller: Roll up and down (a), and sweep the arm (b).

LATISSIMUS DORSI WITH MASSAGE BALL

This technique uses a large massage ball, which is smaller and touches less surface area than a foam roller; therefore, it will apply more pressure.

To begin, lie on your side on a flat, comfortable surface. Stack the legs, and add a slight bend so the hips and knees are relaxed. Then, place the foam roller under the latissimus dorsi, which is about midway up the rib cage, while still sharing some pressure with the shoulder blade. Roll up and down until you find a tender spot and hold (see figure 9.4a). While holding, sweep the arm by reaching the arm directly in front of your body. I typically recommend rotating the shoulder so the palm is facing upward, as it is often more comfortable. Next, keep the muscle pinned and sweep the arm upward, toward your head, until the shoulder is fully flexed (see figure 9.4b). If there is any pain in the shoulder joint while sweeping, then you don't have to go all the way. Only move the shoulder as far as is comfortable, realizing there may naturally be some discomfort from the massage ball.

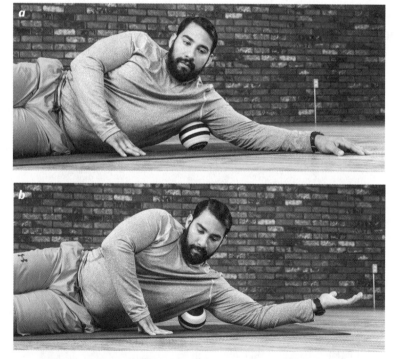

Figure 9.4 Latissimus dorsi with massage ball: Roll up and down *(a)*, and sweep the arm *(b)*.

POSTERIOR DELTOID WITH MASSAGE BALL

There are a few ways to target the posterior deltoid. I suggest performing this release by lying flat on your back on a smooth, comfortable surface, as this position is generally more comfortable and, therefore, more effective. If you need to reduce pressure on the low back, bend the hips and knees so that the feet are flat on the floor. Place the massage ball on the ground, and then position the shoulder on top of it so that the ball is directly behind the shoulder joint. The shoulder will be in a 90-degree position to place the muscle at an optimal length. This technique involves very little rolling, so you will simply find a tender spot and hold (see figure 9.5a). After a period of time or once the tenderness has decreased, move onto shoulder rotations. This movement will apply a slight stretch to the muscle to help it release and lengthen. To perform the rotation, the shoulder should already be out to 90 degrees. Then bend the elbow to 90 degrees so the hand is off the ground. Next, while maintaining pressure, slowly rotate your arm down by lowering your hand toward the ground (see figure 9.5b). Take it only as far as you can while still maintaining pressure on the massage ball.

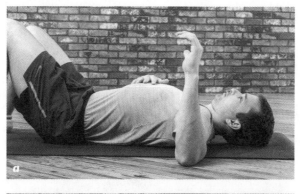

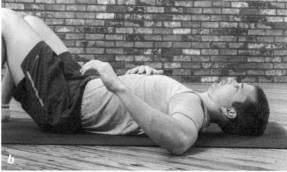

Figure 9.5 Posterior deltoid with massage ball: Hold *(a)* and rotate the arm *(b)*.

LEVATOR SCAPULAE WITH LARGE MASSAGE BALL

Begin by standing near a sturdy wall; about 1 foot, or .3 meters, away is sufficient. Place a large massage ball between the wall and the muscle. The best way to identify the location of the levator scapulae is to reach one hand back to find the tip of the shoulder blade. This inside tip, closer to the spine, is where the levator scapulae begins and is the best place to release the muscle. Once you've reached this spot, lean into the wall; usually this setup position can help you identify the most tender spot; if not, move the ball around to search for a tender spot and hold (see figure 9.6a). If you need more pressure, move the feet further away from the wall. After you've held pressure for a period of time or when the tenderness reduces, move on to the arm raise. This is performed very similarly to the arm sweep in the latissimus dorsi release, except you're standing upright. With the arm relaxed down by your side, raise the arm as high as you can overhead (see figure 9.6b). The same rules apply as far as pain goes: If you have any pain in the shoulder joint, raise as high as you can until the pain begins and stop.

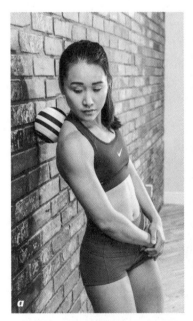 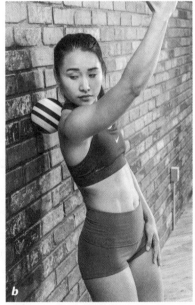

Figure 9.6 Levator scapulae with large massage ball: Hold *(a)* and raise the arm *(b)*.

ARMS

After the areas of the shoulder are addressed, it is now time to move on to the arms. I encourage everyone, even if they have arm pain, to first focus on the muscles that control the shoulders. If the shoulder joint isn't moving well, then the arm is likely taking on additional stress. Therefore, while the arms are important to address, I consider them secondary.

Basic Anatomy of the Arms

This section will focus primarily on the upper arm. This area is relatively simple: It contains the humerus and interacts with both the shoulder and the lower arm at the elbow. Two muscles, the biceps brachii (see figure 9.7a) on the front of the arm and the triceps brachii (see figure 9.7b) on the back of the arm, are relatively simple in design and function. The muscle on the front can bend the elbow and help raise the whole arm. The muscle on the back of the arm extends the elbow and helps to bring the whole arm behind you.

For simplicity, this chapter will refer to the muscles in the forearm as extenders and flexors. The extenders are on the top of the arm and raise the hand up. If you wiggle your fingers, you can see the muscles in this part of the arm move. Therefore, these muscles also help control the fingers. When the wrist is neutral, all of the tendons of the fingers slide through this area with no problems. However, if you were to extend your wrist and then wiggle your fingers, the tendons would have to turn at weird angles to move. While this is not the only cause of wrist problems, this can be an added complication. Therefore, I recommend focusing on the extenders.

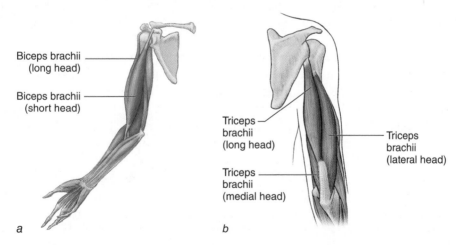

Figure 9.7   Muscles of the upper arms: biceps brachii *(a)* and triceps brachii *(b)*.

Function of the Arms

The function of the arm is relatively simple: It exists so you can feed yourself. Of course, you probably use it to do other tasks, but proper nutrition is vital and the arms are perfectly designed to grab something and bring it to the mouth. In the real world, you may use your arms to carry objects, open doors, and signal nice gestures to a fellow human in traffic. If you really go out of your way to use your arms, maybe you swing from the monkey bars or play by rolling or crawling. Anyone who has ever broke an arm or lost one can attest to the role the arms play in our lives. An arm that is injured or is in chronic pain can wreak havoc on activities of daily living. The muscles of the upper arm, specifically, also help to promote optimal shoulder function. They help move the arm up and down at the shoulder as well as stabilize the shoulder. This is where most of the problems come into play.

Pros and Cons of Rolling the Arms

Rolling the muscles of the arm can help promote ideal function. The most problematic of the arm muscles is the biceps brachii on the front of the upper arm. The biceps don't act alone, however. They typically work to stabilize an unstable shoulder. If they have to work extra hard to do this, a shoulder problem can end up causing a biceps problem. Because of how the biceps attach in the shoulder joint, the biceps can pull the shoulder into a downward position with anterior tipping. (Refer to chapter 8 for a refresher.) One of the most prevalent conditions in the biceps is biceps tendonitis, or inflammation of the tendon of the biceps, commonly due to poor posture. If you have been diagnosed with biceps tendonitis, you may not want to roll the area aggressively. It is already irritated. An easier approach, using a larger and softer foam roller, may work better. A softer roller will promote blood flow and possibly assist in repairing the damaged area.

In the forearm, if the extenders are short and overactive due to chronic wrist extension, this can be deleterious for the tissues that run through the wrist. It also puts extra tension on the elbow, which is the attachment site for the muscles. This pain is commonly called tennis elbow, though it frequently occurs in people who do not play tennis. Using a smaller foam roller or massage ball on these muscles can help to reduce the tension and help increase the ability to stretch them.

In most cases, albeit not all, conditions that affect the arm are secondary. This means that, unless there was a direct impact to the arm or if you play a sport that causes unusual and repetitive forces on the arm, your arm or elbow pain is really caused by poor movement at the shoulder. In my 15 years as a manual therapist and personal trainer, I have assessed thousands of shoulders in people with elbow pain; more than half have had a shoulder limitation that was causing abnormal stress down the rest of the arm. If you are having elbow pain even after treating the site of the pain, consult with a health care provider.

The wrist is similar in that conditions are often secondary; however, many people who frequently use a keyboard experience more direct carpal tunnel, arising from the chronic extended position of the wrists. Foam rolling some of the areas around the wrist alleviate some discomfort, but a change in workplace ergonomics is in order for a long-term fix. As I type these words, I am using a keyboard that elevates my wrists approximately 2 inches, or 5.1 centimeters, off the desk. Thus, my wrist is in a completely neutral position, which does not abnormally compress any nerves or arteries. A keyboard such as this may take some time to get used to, but it is definitely worth it in the end.

Foam Rolling Techniques for the Arms

To begin, slowly roll the area at a tempo of about 1 inch, or 2.5 centimeters, per second to identify any tender spots. A tender spot is something you identify as being painful or uncomfortable. As a general rule of thumb, on a scale of 1 (no pain) to 10 (worst pain imaginable), search for a spot that feels somewhere between a 5 and an 8. Less than a 5 may not be enough discomfort to encourage change, and any spots with pain greater than an 8 may involve too much pain to allow change. These tender spots may indicate that some type of adhesion, knot, or trigger point is present.

Once a spot is identified, relax the muscle that is being rolled and simply breathe into it. This should generally last for 30 to 60 seconds or until you feel a reduction in tenderness; then, add small motions. While each of these additional motions will be different depending on the body part being rolled, most will follow the same pattern of trying to "pin and stretch" the muscle. You can do this by holding pressure and moving a joint close to the roller. Never roll up and down as quickly as possible.

Before you begin, please remember that if you have a medically diagnosed condition, you should not try to go as deep as possible (unless you are under the supervision of your health care provider). Additionally, there is nothing wrong with foam rolling the other muscles of the arm. It is usually the biceps and the forearm extenders that contribute to arm problems, so they are included in this section.

FRONT OF ARM WITH FOAM ROLLER

The bicep can be sufficiently addressed with a regular-sized foam roller. This is one of the easiest and most comfortable releases in the whole book. Begin by lying face down. I would suggest you place the arm that is not being rolled on the ground, so the head can relax on it. To find a tender spot, you will have to move your body side to side on the roller. The tender areas of this muscle are usually found closer to the shoulder. Once you find a tender spot, hold pressure on it (see figure 9.8a). After enough time has passed or when you feel a reduction in tenderness, move on to the cross-friction. Perform the cross-friction by moving the arm up and down and dragging it across the roller (see figure 9.8b). This motion usually doesn't require a lot of motion, as the goal is to get that simple dragging force across the muscle fibers.

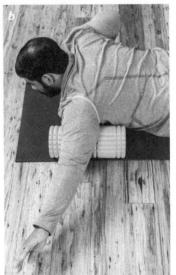

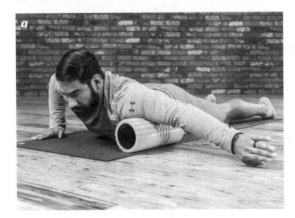

Figure 9.8 Front of arm with foam roller: Hold *(a)* and move the arm up and down *(b)*.

FRONT OF ARM WITH LARGE MASSAGE BALL

When using a massage ball on the bicep, a larger ball usually works better. It is often too difficult to get enough pressure with a smaller ball. This, again, is a very comfortable release. Begin by lying face down and resting the head on the arm that is not being rolled. Then, move your body side to side to find a tender spot. Once you find it, hold pressure on it (see figure 9.9a). The tender areas of this muscle are usually found closer to the shoulder. After enough time has passed or when you feel a reduction in tenderness, move on to the cross-friction. Perform the cross-friction by moving the arm up and down and dragging it across the massage ball (see figure 9.9b). This motion usually doesn't require a lot of motion, as the goal is to get that simple dragging force across the muscle fibers.

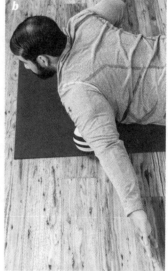

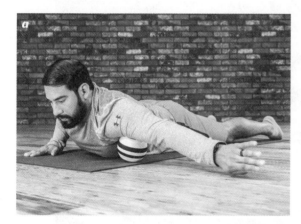

Figure 9.9 Front of arm with large massage ball: Hold *(a)* and move the arm up and down *(b)*.

FOREARM EXTENDERS WITH MASSAGE BALL

The release for the forearm may be performed on a massage ball of any size; however, a smaller massage ball is typically more effective. This release is better if performed either at a desk or, if you're in a gym, on an exercise bench. Begin by positioning yourself in front of the desk or bench. Then, place the massage ball on the surface, and place the back of the forearm on top of the massage ball. Use the hand that is not being rolled to apply additional pressure if needed. Begin near the wrist, and roll toward the elbow until you find a tender spot. Once you find a spot, hold pressure while fully rolling the wrist (see figure 9.10a) and then fully flexing it (see figure 9.10b).

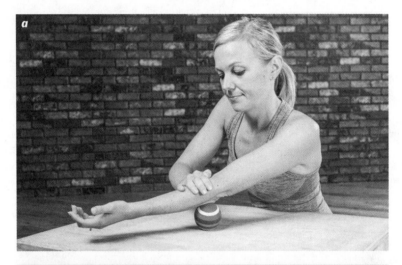

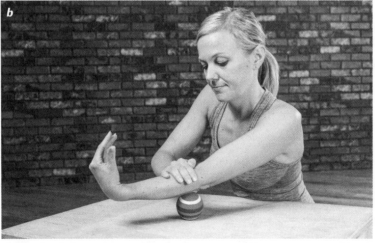

Figure 9.10 Forearm extenders with massage ball: Hold, then roll the wrist *(a)*, and flex the wrist *(b)*.

FOREARM FLEXORS WITH MASSAGE BALL

You will perform this technique exactly like the previous technique, except you will place the opposite muscle on the massage ball. Begin by positioning yourself in front of the table or bench. Then, place the massage ball on the surface, and place the front of the forearm on top of the massage ball. Use the hand that is not being rolled to apply additional pressure if needed. Begin near the wrist, and roll toward the elbow until you find a tender spot. Once you find one, hold pressure and roll the wrist (see figure 9.11a) and then fully extend it (see figure 9.11b).

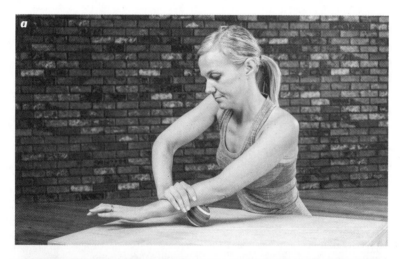

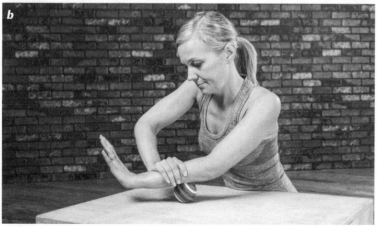

Figure 9.11 Forearm flexors with massage ball: Hold, then roll the wrist *(a)*, and extend the wrist *(b)*.

The muscles in and around the shoulder and arm can play a part in many different types of dysfunction, from shoulder impingement to tennis elbow. However, these muscles usually work, albeit incorrectly, with many other parts of the body. Therefore, it is imperative to also roll the areas of the chest and upper back to get the most benefit from the shoulder and arm releases.

Part III

PROGRAMMING

Chapter 10

FULL-BODY ASSESSMENT

One of the biggest mistakes people make in health and fitness is not knowing where to begin. It's like having a map. You may have the best directions in the world, but if you don't have a starting point, then you may not reach your destination. Most people begin foam rolling by following whatever others are doing at the gym or by simply rolling the areas of the body that hurt or feel tight. However, it's important to get to the root of the problem if you want to change it.

The late Professor Shirley Sahrmann once remarked that we confuse tightness with stiffness. In her 2002 book, she suggested that a muscle that feels tight is rarely short and tight; rather, it is stiff or simply does not shorten and lengthen the way it should. There is nothing wrong with foam rolling areas that you think need it. However, if you have an issue, such as nagging low back pain, then you must do something to figure out exactly which muscles need which solution. Some muscles need foam rolling and stretching, while others likely need strengthening. This chapter will teach you how to perform a movement assessment on yourself and to provide insight into your flexibility and which muscles you need to target to improve it.

PERFORMING A MOVEMENT ASSESSMENT

In a keynote address at the International Federation of Orthopedic Manipulative Physical Therapist convention in 2012, physical therapist Gray Cook said, "Look for signs before symptoms; we must identify faulty function, and we have to change it" (Cook, 2012). Cook developed a series of tests to help identify the root cause of movement dysfunction. These tests were designed for fitness professionals to use on their clients. This book will not incorporate Cook's tests, but it is worth researching further if you are interested.

To assess your flexibility and strength, this chapter will employ a simple squat. The squat test is part of Cook's screening, and the National Academy of Sports Medicine also uses the squat as one of their primary assessments. Performing a squat with the arms overhead (overhead squat) provides a quick snapshot of how the body moves overall. Of course, one movement doesn't reveal all information, but it will begin to point you in the right direction.

To squat correctly, the body must demonstrate appropriate levels of flexibility and strength. An ideal squat will require the following:

- ~20 degrees of movement at the ankle
- ~120 degrees of movement at the knee
- ~120 degrees of movement at the hip
- ~180 degrees of movement at the shoulder

More joints could be measured, but these are the main joints that, if altered, lead to problems in other areas. For example, if the ankle couldn't move during a squat, pressure would increase in the hip and low back. Thus, tight calves, which limit ankle motion, can be a factor in low back pain. Additionally, many muscles influence these four joints. Therefore, all foam rolling (and probably any stretch you've ever done in your life) has something to do with these joints.

The overhead squat assessment can be used as a snapshot of movement quality. Additional tests can help determine exactly what is going on in the body. However, these usually take a considerable amount of training and skill and should be performed by a licensed practitioner.

Squat Assessment Checkpoints

Squatting is a movement that all humans do, even when they do not realize it. However, the squat is often performed improperly. A key factor in using the squat as an assessment is making sure it is set up correctly. If you were to take 100 people and ask them to squat, you would probably see 90 different squats. Of course, everyone moves slightly differently. However, research has suggested a few checkpoints in the body are highly associated with injury. These checkpoints are as follows.

Straight Feet

The foot is not designed to function with the toes out like a duck (see figure 10.1a) but with the toes pointing straight ahead (see figure 10.1b). The design functions like a suspension bridge. When you walk, run, lunge, or squat, this design helps support the foot. If the foot does not have adequate support, the most common method of compensation in the foot and ankle is to turn the feet outward when walking and squatting. This alters the entire biomechanics of the foot and lower leg, sets the stage for problems like plantar fasciitis,

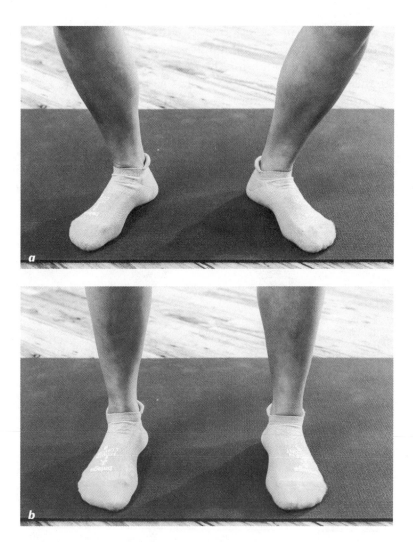

Figure 10.1 Foot position for a squat: incorrect *(a)* and correct *(b)*.

and does not help those with chronic ankle sprains. Now, if you are squatting to set a world record in weightlifting, you may turn your feet out to increase the base of support and allow more weight to be moved. However, the norm for the foot should be to point straight. This might feel strange because the muscles in this area have likely shortened to support your walking patterns—just because the position is the norm doesn't mean it's ideal. Your goal should be to return to the ideal position, where the joints have the least amount of stress and injuries are less prevalent.

Aligned Knees

The knee (more specifically, the patella) is designed to track in line with the foot. This is actually one of the more researched aspects of the squat assessment.

If the knee moves either inside or outside of the foot, then the chance of knee injuries increase. Researchers Bell, Padua, and Clark (2008) found that if the knee moves inward far enough for the patella to track inside of the big toe, then the chances of a knee injury increases significantly. The knees moving inward is a common compensation largely due to the function of the foot and the hip. However, while less common, the knees moving outward too far (see figure 10.2a) can also lead to knee problems. Therefore, during a squat, the knee should track in line with the foot (see figure 10.2b). Additionally, the old adage that the knees cannot go past the toes is based on old research. New research suggests the knees may go past the toes as long as they don't move inward or outward too far.

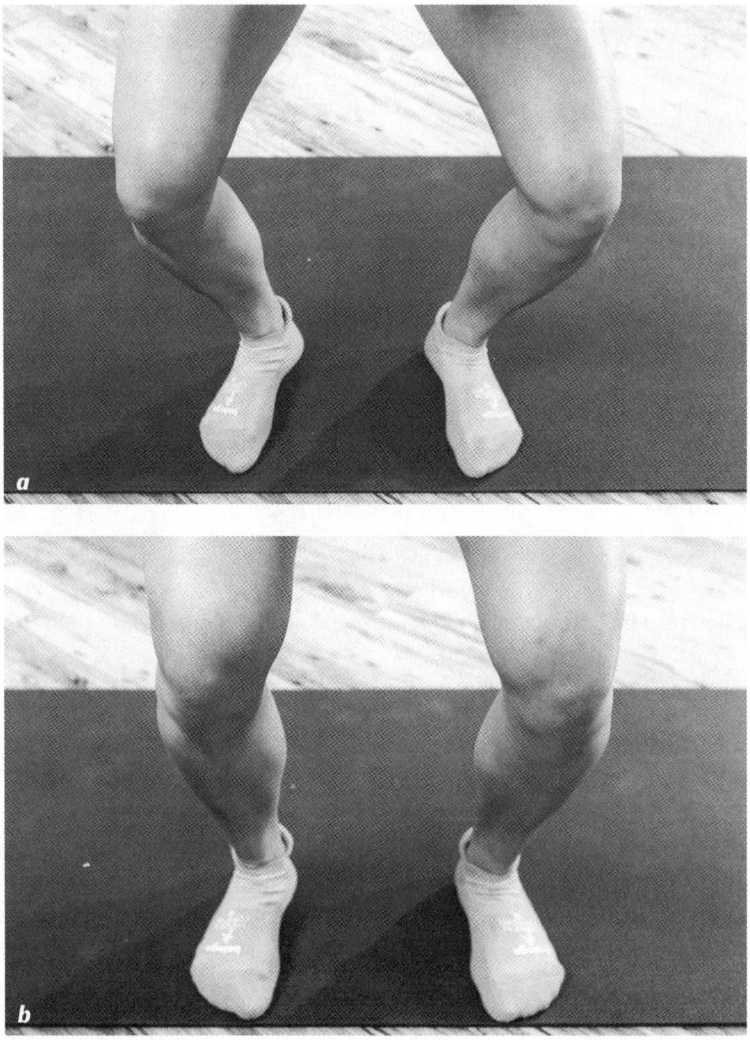

Figure 10.2 Knee alignment for a squat: incorrect *(a)* and correct *(b)*.

Neutral Pelvis

The ability of the pelvis to stay neutral has a lot to do with not only the health of the hip joint but also the low back. Because of the way the spine connects to the pelvis, if the pelvis moves, then the lumbar spine moves, too. Therefore, if you keep the pelvis neutral during a squat, the lumbar spine will also remain neutral, lowering the likelihood of injury or chronic pain. Two positions in the squat assessment can indicate an individual is more at risk of low back pain. The most common is the anterior pelvic tilt (see figure 10.3a). This is very common in today's population because people are seated more often and because of the way people walk and for many other reasons. This position places additional, unnecessary stress on the tissue of the low back and can lead to problems. During a squat, the pelvis and spine should remain neutral, whatever neutral is to you (see figure 10.3b). One simple way to identify neutral is simply to tilt your pelvis forward as far as you can. (Imagine your hips are a bucket of water and you're pouring the water out of the front of the bucket.) Then, tilt the pelvis back as far as you can (imagine you're pouring the water out of the back). Finally, move somewhere in the middle of those two points. This can be considered your neutral. The goal is now to maintain neutral during the squat. If the pelvis tilts in any direction, then it simply means there is an area of opportunity for the muscles around the hips.

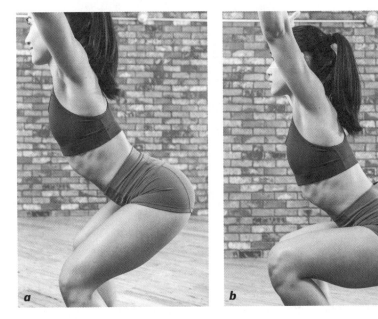

Figure 10.3 Pelvis position for a squat: incorrect (a) and correct (b).

Parallel Torso

With the body proportioned the way it is, ideal form usually produces nice, congruent angles. During a squat, when the ankle, knee, and hip all move optimally, the knee and the hip are positioned at equal angles. If one of these joints doesn't move the way it is supposed to, the tibia (lower leg) and torso are unable to maintain parallel (see figure 10.4a). Rather, the tibia and torso must maintain parallel lines throughout the motion (see figure 10.4b).

It should be noted that the lines between the tibia and torso aren't always parallel during exercise. For example, a deadlift (which is probably one of the most valuable moves in exercise) occurs when you let the torso move forward (bending at the hip) while ensuring the knees don't bend more than a few degrees. However, if you can't squat with parallel lines, this indicates room for improvement. Think of all the times you perform a squat motion using the restroom, getting in and out of a car, sitting for dinner, and so on. Over time, if the squat is performed repeatedly without parallel lines, it may increase the pressure to the low back.

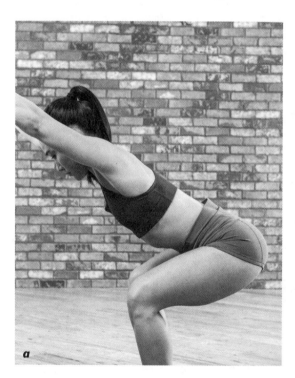 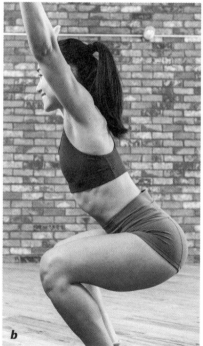

Figure 10.4 Torso position for a squat: incorrect *(a)* and correct *(b)*.

Arms Overhead and Aligned

For many people, simply raising their arms completely overhead is hard enough—much less having the strength in the muscles around the shoulder blade to keep the arms raised during a squat. This is a red flag: If the muscles around your shoulder are so inflexible that they can't demonstrate the full range of motion, then it is likely you already have a shoulder injury or may have one soon. This motion, called shoulder flexion, requires the shoulder muscles to lengthen. When raising the arms overhead, it is important to keep the spine neutral. If you arch the lower back in order to get the arms up, you must compensate at the pelvis to add additional motion to the shoulder. While this may protect the shoulder in the short term, it will lead to low back problems or shoulder problems in the long term. During a squat, the arms should not fall forward (see figure 10.5*a*). Rather, the arms should remain in line with the torso (see figure 10.5*b*).

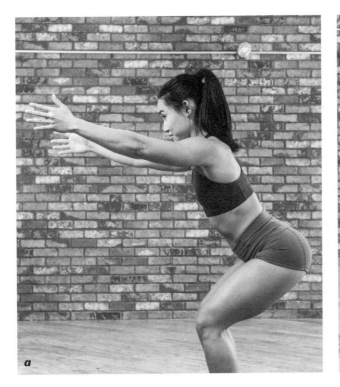 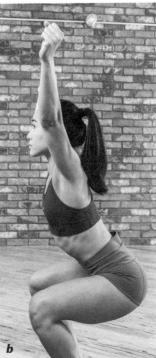

Figure 10.5 Arm position for a squat: incorrect *(a)* and correct *(b)*.

Completing Your Squat Assessment

The overhead squat assessment is easy to perform on yourself as long as you have a full-length mirror. If not, then have a friend take a video of you performing the assessment. I recommend performing this without shoes. Shoes often provide support—which is great for long walks but not so great when you need to see how the body works. Two exceptions are as follows: (1) if you are in a setting, such as a gym, that prohibits you from removing your shoes or (2) if you have prescription orthotics that a physician is requiring you to wear. Over-the-counter Dr. Scholl's® inserts do not count—only orthotics that were prescribed by your physician and built for you.

Begin by standing tall with your feet approximately hip or shoulder-width apart. As mentioned earlier, while it may seem more comfortable to stand with the feet wider, it makes the assessment less effective and isn't as natural as you might think. Both feet need to be parallel and pointing straight ahead. Assume the same stance during the squat that you might assume when skiing. The knee caps should point in the same direction as the feet. The hips can be set to your neutral by placing your hands on your hips, tilting the pelvis forward as far as you can, and then tilting them back as far as you can (finally settling somewhere in between). Then, reach the arms overhead. Now, perform 5 to 10 squats, pressing the gluteals down so the thighs are parallel and coming back up at a comfortable pace. See figure 10.6 for an example of a properly executed squat.

You don't have to be perfect, but be sure you challenge yourself to squat to that depth. It is not necessary, for assessment purposes, to go any lower. However, frequently people will squat down only as far as they can *before* they compensate. While this may be safe, it is unrealistic. In life, you sometimes have to squat lower than you might like. You likely already experience a squat depth, where the thighs are parallel, when you move on and off of a toilet. If you compensate in this overhead squat assessment, it is a guarantee that you probably compensate during any other stand-to-sit or sit-to-stand movements. Accumulation of the compensation over time leads to injury. If you feel pain at any point during the squat, make a note of it. If the pain is too much for you to continue, consult with your physician. However, if you feel comfortable continuing with the overhead squat assessment, then feel free to do so. View yourself from two different views, a front view and a side view.

Front View

Begin by looking directly into the mirror. From this view, check to see if your feet stay straight or turn out and whether your knees stay aligned. If they don't, it simply means that some foam rolling and stretching may do you good. You'll need to consider what type of surface you're on as you are squatting. If you are standing on a rubber floor, such as a gym floor, there is a good chance that your feet will stick to it. You may want to find a hard-

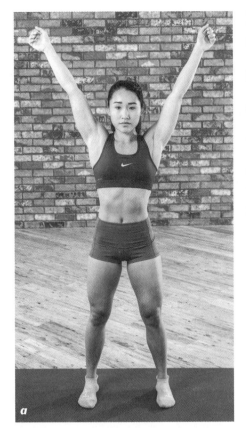 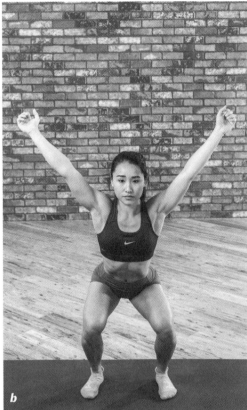

Figure 10.6 Properly executed squat.

wood floor and wear socks. A slightly slippery surface will allow you to see the compensations better.

Side View

Now, turn 90 degrees to get a side view. This one will be more challenging to do alone, but you can turn your head as you squat to check out what is happening. Be sure you realign your feet and knees. Many times when people rotate, they spread their feet out to go back to where they are comfortable. A wide stance will make it easier to squat, and you won't be able to see the compensation that may lead to injury someday. Again, repeat the process of squatting down to where the thighs are approximately parallel, and perform 5 to 10 squats. Try to first see if your spine is staying neutral or if it is arching. Then try to notice if the torso and tibia (lower leg) are close to parallel or if the torso is caving in on the lower body. Lastly, from the side view, try to see what the arms are doing. Are they staying overhead or falling forward? Many times people will move their arms all around during the squat. However, during the overhead squat assessment, they need to remain stationary.

When assessing yourself, it may help to make a chart for notes and reminders of what to examine. You can Google charts online, create your own, or use the chart provided here (see figure 10.7). Check "yes" or "no" in the boxes to designate where you have movement compensations.

	Compensation	Yes or No?	Comments/Notes
Front View	Feet Out		
	Knees In		
Side View	Anterior Pelvic Tilt		
	Excessive Forward Lean		
	Arms Forward		

Figure 10.7 Squat assessment checklist.
From K. Stull, 2018, *Complete guide to foam rolling* (Champaign, IL: Human Kinetics).

INTERPRETING YOUR RESULTS

Once you've completed the overhead squat assessment and jotted down your findings, it's then time to figure out what to do with that information. The movement compensations listed in figure 10.7 can be traced back to a couple of muscle groups that have been discussed in previous chapters. The following list will tell you which muscle groups to foam roll and direct you to the specific chapter so you can review further if needed.

Feet Turn Out

The feet turn out, in most cases, when the muscles that cross the ankle joint shortened. If these muscle lack proper extensibility, then the body has to move around that joint. Therefore, if this is your primary compensation, foam roll:

- Bottom of the foot (chapter 5)
- Calves (chapter 5)

Knees Move In

When the knees cave in, this compensation is generally a combination of issues with both the ankle and the hip (the knee is simply the connection located between those two joints). Therefore, if this is your primary compensation, foam roll:

- Calves (chapter 5)
- Quadriceps (chapter 6)
- Adductors (chapter 6)
- Tensor fascia latae or TFL (chapter 7)
- Piriformis (chapter 7)

Anterior Pelvic Tilt

The pelvic tilt compensation occurs frequently among people who spend most of their day seated (which is most people). During a seated position, the muscles in the front of the hip shorten, while the muscles in the back of the hip lengthen. After too long, it is easier for the body to adapt to this position than it is for the body to attempt to lengthen those areas. Additionally, one of the muscles of the upper body attaches to the back of the pelvis and contributes to this movement pattern. Therefore, if this is your primary compensation, foam roll:

- Quadriceps (chapter 6)
- TFL (chapter 7)
- Piriformis (chapter 7)
- Latissimus dorsi (chapter 9)

Excessive Forward Lean

If the torso is leaning forward excessively, this compensation usually means the body needs to maintain its center of gravity. In most cases, this occurs when the calves have lost flexibility. However, a few muscles around the hips could be contributing to the issue. Therefore, if this is your primary compensation, foam roll:

- Calves (chapter 5)
- Quadriceps (chapter 6)
- TFL (chapter 7)

Arms Fall Forward

Last, but certainly not least, is the compensation in which the arms fall forward. The muscles of the chest and back pull down on the arm, most often the result of a faulty movement pattern. However, a stiff upper back could also prevent the arms from making overhead. Therefore, if this is your primary movement compensation, foam roll:

- Thoracic spine (chapter 8)
- Pectorals (chapter 8)
- Latissimus dorsi (chapter 9)

You probably noticed that several muscle groups showed up more than once in the assessment while others mentioned in this book didn't make the list at all. First, the areas that show up more than once are areas that are more likely to be dysfunctional in most people. These include the calves, quadriceps, piriformis, and latissimus dorsi. It is safe to assume that almost anyone could benefit from foam rolling those areas on a daily basis. You will notice some muscles didn't make the list at all, such as the levator scapulae, the biceps, and the triceps. This doesn't mean they aren't important. It simply means that fewer issues arise with these areas, or they are harder to test. If you recall, the levator scapulae (discussed in chapter 9) is part of the shoulder and is near sensitive areas in the neck. It is not bad to roll the levator scapulae; however, if you are having neck pain, it is better to consult with your physician before trying to roll it. Additionally, many of the muscles of the arms (discussed in chapter 9) don't show up on this list. Again, they are great to roll but to identify them as a factor in a movement problem takes more specific testing, which is outside the scope of this book.

Lastly, you may have demonstrated more than just one of the movement compensations above. As you see, many of the muscles cross over into multiple compensations. The calves, for example, show up in three of the different faulty patterns. You don't have to roll everything every day. Instead, prioritize the foam rolling by rolling the worst area and the second to worst area. Then, foam roll the muscles that contribute to the worst movement three days a week, and roll the secondary muscles two days a week. Give yourself one day off for good behavior.

Foam rolling can serve many great purposes, from improving performance to reducing soreness and speeding up recovery. However, to get the most out of your foam rolling, use movement assessments for programming guidance. The overhead squat assessment will provide insight into how your body moves and what you can do to maintain or improve ideal movement. This will help you achieve results much more quickly.

Chapter 11

WARM-UP

A proper warm-up is essential for safety and optimal performance before athletic activity. Warming up is not complicated, but it is often misunderstood. The key is not necessarily to increase body temperature but to introduce movement to all of the sliding surfaces in the body. The risk of pulling a muscle increases when it isn't able to relax and contract accordingly. Additionally, a warm-up doesn't take place only before sporting events. You could use a warm-up before you sit at a desk all day. Sitting applies abnormal stress on the body and may cause just as many injuries as athletic events. One of the best ways to warm up, for whatever activity, is by foam rolling. The compression and the techniques discussed in previous chapters will increase the body's ability to move fluently, thereby decreasing the abnormal stresses applied during activity or sitting. This chapter will discuss how foam rolling prior to your activity will best prepare you to move well and demonstrate adequate strength.

BENEFITS OF FOAM ROLLING PRIOR TO ACTIVITY

Chapter 1 explained much of the current literature surrounding foam rolling. Several of those studies set out to determine the foam roller's role in a warm-up by rolling prior to physical activity. As a brief review, one study found that foam rolling before testing jump height may increase the ability to jump, while others suggested that foam rolling may increase the ability to contract muscles. Another study demonstrated that foam rolling prior to activity may reduce the feelings of fatigue. Other studies found that foam rolling increases flexibility and range of motion without negatively affecting performance. This is important to some sporting populations because certain types of stretching may negatively affect performance. Studies have found improved blood flow in the upper leg after foam rolling only the lower leg. These findings coincide with the suggestion that foam rolling prior to activity may reduce the chance of injury. While there have been no long-term studies on foam rolling and injury to date, short-term studies suggest that increasing blood flow and improving overall mobility will decrease the chance of sustaining common overuse injuries. I do believe this to be true.

A "warm-up" is defined as preparing for physical activity, and the true value of a warm-up is its ability to increase blood flow to the areas of the body that are going to be used most. A typical warm-up before activity involves, in many cases, performing the exact same activity but at a lower level of intensity. While this is not entirely wrong, it may not get the blood flowing or prepare the tissues for activity. This is where foam rolling can have a positive effect. Foam rolling applies compression directly to the muscles, which will encourage blood flow throughout the body. Therefore, the National Academy of Sports Medicine, TriggerPoint, and other credible organizations suggest using foam rolling at the beginning of the warm-up and as part of what is frequently called "movement prep." Movement prep involves a variety of stretching techniques, should be based on the movement assessment, and changes over time.

As discussed in chapter 10, you should foam roll areas based on how you move and not necessarily how you feel or what you do—although, if you move well and feel well, you can roll whatever areas you want. If you're dealing with aches and pains, then use the assessment in chapter 10 as a guide. There are no exact sport specific programs to follow since the ideal program is based on how you move. Generally, foam rolling programs should be human-specific. This means that all humans should meet certain movement parameters. If they don't, regardless of sport, their risk of injury increases. This means that there are no magical areas that all runners need to roll. Likewise, cycling on the weekends doesn't prequalify you to perform special rolling techniques. However, many runners suffer from the same injuries, and cycling on the weekends may change your movement in specific ways. Therefore, this chapter will provide some general guidelines as a starting point for foam rolling.

After working in the health and fitness industry for 13 years and having a firm understanding of the principles of human movement, I have found there are areas that frequently need attention. Cassidy Phillips, founder of Trigger-Point, suggested that most people need to concentrate on six primary areas (the "Ultimate Six"):

- Soleus muscle of the lower leg
- Quadriceps of the upper leg
- Piriformis deep in the hip
- Psoas in the abdominal region

- Thoracic spine of the upper back
- Pectorals of the chest

After years of case studies, these six problem areas do indeed show up in many active people. (The one exception that does not appear to be as dysfunctional as most people think is the psoas.) Surprisingly, many athletes suffer from similar injuries, the majority of which are overuse or repetitive movement injuries. What may also seem unusual is that many of the same injuries that occur in a sedentary individual may be seen in a competitive athlete. Therefore, no matter your sport or activity of choice, it is likely that you will be rolling many of the Ultimate Six muscles often.

One thing to consider before moving on is an injury sustained during a contact sport. If a linebacker smacks you in the side of the knee, you will likely experience an injury. No amount of foam rolling can prevent contact injuries.

WARM-UP GUIDELINES FOR SPECIFIC SPORTS AND GENERAL ACTIVITIES

Any type of activity can place stress on the body. Stress is a good thing because it encourages the body to adapt. However, too much stress or stress focused too much in one area of the body will lead to overuse and eventual injury. Many of the injuries suffered in sports can be traced back to overuse. It's not that the body can't handle the stress but that the specific foot, knee, or hip is taking on much more stress than it should. This next section will discuss some of the most common athletic and lifestyle activities and will suggest some key muscle groups to roll for the optimal warm-up.

Running

Running is one of the most popular athletic activities in the world. A recent trends study suggested gym memberships are decreasing while participation in cross-country sports is increasing (ACSM, 2016). This is great news because the human body is made to run. However, when the body is tight, stiff, or simply not functioning optimally, running can wreak havoc on the knees, hips, and low back. I often hear long-time runners saying, "My knees are bad because I'm a runner." They believe that the impact and pounding over the years has caused problems. In fact, it's not the running that has caused the problem but the way they ran. One study published in the *Journal of Sports Sciences* suggested that people who run with optimal form experience little increase in impact, whereas poor form increases forces as much as 33 times the body weight at the knee (Harrison et al., 1986). Therefore, if you want to be a long-term runner, make sure your running mechanics are sound. Seek out a running coach or personal trainer who has studied running. Even if you're a "weekend warrior," spending a little time and money learning the correct way to run could save you thousands on a knee replacement later in life.

Foam rolling the following four areas as part of your warm-up may help to improve running mechanics. Remember, the best results come from performing an assessment.

- Calves
- Tensor fascia latae (TFL)
- Vastus lateralis
- Thoracic spine

Cycling

Cycling is a great low-impact sport that can be exhilarating and effective for people with weight loss goals who are already dealing with aches and pains. However, surprisingly, one of the most common complaints in cycling is knee pain, and most people believe the cause is overuse. However, much like we see in running, the knee is made to move in the exact motion used in cycling. Thus, overuse doesn't make much sense. What does make sense, however, is poor mechanics. Many cyclists have massive upper leg muscles and calves. These look great, but if they get too tight or short, they will alter mechanics, leading to excessive wear and tear at the surrounding joints. To properly prepare the lower body for cycling, begin by foam rolling the following areas:

- Calves
- Quadriceps
- Hamstrings

Many cyclists also suffer from upper body aches and pains. It is common for someone to experience low back pain and neck tension while riding. These aches have a slightly different cause than the knee pain. The aerodynamic position created during riding puts the low back in a flexed position. While the low back can easily flex, flexing the low back for hours and hours per day is the one of the leading causes of back pain. The pain may not be caused solely by cycling but is likely an accumulation of stress to the low back from cycling and then sitting throughout the day. In addition, when in the aerodynamic position, the head is up so the eyes can see forward. In most cases, I recommend exercises to keep a neutral neck position. However, when speeding down the street on a bike, you need to look where you're going. Again, over time, this is likely to lead to neck tension and pain. As a rehabilitation specialist, when people come to me with this issue, I must inform them that their activity of choice may not be causing the pain, but it's certainly not helping. I have worked with far too many athletes who love their sport to give it up or even take much time off. Therefore, foam rolling the following areas as part of a daily warm-up may help to reduce some of the discomfort, but it is not likely going to totally eliminate or prevent it:

- Thoracic spine
- Pectorals
- Upper trapezius

Swimming

Swimming requires amazing athletics, regardless of whether the swimmer is a professional or an enthusiast. The coordination of movement and breathing during swimming is something that few have mastered. A comprehensive study published in the *American Journal of Sports Medicine* found that elite swimmers sustained approximately four injuries for every 1,000 training sessions (Wolf et al., 2009). Shoulder injuries are the most common, with more than 90 percent of athlete swimmers dealing with shoulder pain at some point. This comes as no surprise, considering the hours of training and the amount of movement and force produced by the shoulder during competition. When muscles in the chest and back shorten and are overactive, due to overuse or being sedentary, they can pull on the shoulder in ways that begin to limit full range of motion. However, to swim correctly requires all available motion. Many of the shoulder injuries sustained during swimming are likely due to forcing motion on an area that has become restricted. To prevent a shoulder injury, or if you have already sustained one, foam roll the following areas before swimming:

- Thoracic spine
- Pectorals
- Latissimus dorsi

Surprisingly, knee injuries are the second most common injury in swimming, followed closely by low back pain. Kaneoka et al. (2007) found that out of 56 elite swimmers, 68% of them suffered from degenerative disc disease. This was primarily seen at the disc between the last lumbar spine and the sacrum, which is a common site for back pain. These percentages are too high to be coincidence. However, as with most sports, someone passionate about swimming isn't going to give up their sport over a few aches and pains. I don't support the "no pain, no gain" attitude, as pain hurts for a reason: Your body wants you to stop or try a different technique. Nevertheless, if you insist on continuing, add the following to your warm-up routine to ease or prevent knee or low back pain:

- Quadriceps
- Adductors
- Iliotibial (IT) band

Hiking

Hiking is an activity that few people relate to injury—unless you are a hiker. Sustaining an injury while hiking could be the start of a terrible day. Many hikers travel deep into dangerous territory or hike up mountains and hills that can quickly see drastic changes in weather. The ability to move quickly to safety could save someone's life. The most common injury experienced by hikers is an ankle sprain. In many cases, ankle sprains are considered a non-contact injury, thus avoidable. However, given that hiking involves moving across slippery rocks or trails with deep crevices, the injury may be classified as a "contact" injury, or at least as unavoidable. There is no proven way to protect yourself against slipping on a rock and twisting an ankle. However, if the ankle and entire lower extremity receives more blood flow and has received a thorough warm-up, the severity of the injury may be decreased when sustained. Before you hike, take five minutes to roll the following areas:

- Feet
- Calves
- Quadriceps
- Adductors
- Hamstrings
- Hips

Weightlifting

The most common injuries sustained during weight training or weightlifting are overuse injuries. Keep in mind, an overuse injury is largely preventable. A great warm-up, for example, may help to reduce the chance of sustaining such an injury. The top injuries in weightlifting are shoulder injuries (including shoulder impingement and rotator cuff tears), patellar tendonitis, and back sprains and strains. Shoulder impingement is extremely common and in many cases is related to poor posture or poor weightlifting form. Similarly, back sprains and strains could be related to the poor posture seen in many sedentary individuals who then try to place too much load on the back. If you have any questions about your posture or weightlifting form, speak to a certified personal trainer before beginning a weight training program.

Remember that an ideal foam rolling program should be based on how you move and not on how you feel. Perform a movement assessment, and then foam roll the following muscle groups as part of your warm-up to prevent weightlifting injuries:

- Calves
- Quadriceps
- Hips
- Thoracic spine
- Pectorals
- Latissimus dorsi

Cross-Training

Cross-training is quite simply the most popular form of training or exercise. It is defined as training in two or more sports in order to improve fitness or performance. Thus, cross-training could combine weightlifting and running. In my professional opinion, everyone should always be cross-training. One of the main reasons for injuries is overuse. The body is made to be used, but it is also made for variety. Repetitive movement leads to overuse injuries. If you're a runner, for example, running is causing your body stress—good stress that the body must be given time to repair and recover. If you're a cross-trainer, you could let your body recover from running while you perform a different activity like snow skiing (anything that involves a pattern different than running). However, do not assume anything different is advantageous. Running and cycling, while different in nature, involve a similar pattern for the body. The ankles, knees, and hips are performing almost the exact same movement in both activities. Therefore, to truly see the benefits of cross-training, running should not be paired with cycling. The patterns are just too similar. Try something with a different pattern such as in-line skating, ice-skating, dancing, or weight training with total body movements.

Since cross-training involves a combination of activities, it makes sense to roll a combination of areas. Here is a list of areas to roll—keep in mind that the assessment should be your guide:

- Calves
- Quadriceps
- Hips
- Thoracic spine
- Pectorals

Sitting at a Desk

The U.S. Department of Labor (2015) suggested that 32 percent of all workplace injuries in 2014 were musculoskeletal injuries. They define musculoskeletal injuries as any injury or disorder to the soft tissues (muscles, tendons, ligaments, and joints). Most of the injuries presented in the arms and back. Not only does this cost the workplace in lost productivity, but also this has a negative impact on morale. This book is not a replacement for a comprehensive corporate wellness program, but foam rolling the following areas several times throughout the workday may help to reduce many discomforts associated with being sedentary all day:

- Hips
- Hamstrings
- Thoracic spine
- Pectorals
- Latissimus dorsi

Managing Low Back Pain

So far this chapter has primarily discussed the areas of the body to roll before participating in athletic events. However, many people dealing with certain conditions need to simply prepare the muscles for daily life. For example, low back pain affects more than 80 percent of the population and, in most cases, cannot be attributed to any specific event. Therefore, low back pain is often considered an overuse injury. When certain muscles are pulling on the hips and other muscles are not able to support them, the structures of the low back pay the price. Low back pain can be related to many issues, so if you're dealing with significant pain be sure to speak with your physician before foam rolling. If you are able to begin a foam rolling program, start by rolling the following muscles. While these muscles may not appear to directly affect the low back, they do play a role in overall biomechanics. The biomechanics of low back pain begin at the ground. If the ankle doesn't move optimally, there is a chance that too much load will be placed on the joints above. So, begin at the ground and work up in the following areas:

- Calves
- Quadriceps
- Hips
- Thoracic spine

Common areas of confusion for low back pain is the low back itself and the hamstrings. The low back does not inflict pain on itself. In fact, it usually tightens in order to protect itself. Therefore, rolling the low back may provide short-term relief but will not get to the root of the problem. The same may be said for the hamstrings. They are often tight in those suffering with low back pain. However, they are usually tense and stiff and not actually tight and short. Foam rolling the hamstrings will likely not hurt anything, but again, it's not getting to the root of the problem. I encourage you to spend two to three weeks just working on mobility for the muscles listed in this section. For additional exercise, work on core stabilization exercises. This would include exercises such as glute bridges (to strengthen the hips) and planks (to strengthen the core muscles).

Preventing Injury

Ideally, we would all continuously work to prevent injuries before they occur. This is not always doable, of course, but is a great mindset. Certain injuries, such as shoulder injuries, not only are painful, but also are incredibly difficult to get under control. Some estimates suggest that more than 25 percent of the U.S. population is currently dealing with a shoulder injury, and more than 40 percent of those with shoulder pain have it for more than two years. Therefore, the best thing you can do for a shoulder injury is to prevent it from ever happening. This is the case for all injuries, as one of the best predictors of an injury is a past injury. The best injury prevention plan is one that is based on the movement assessment. However, if for some reason you are unable to perform an assessment, you can still foam roll the following areas to prepare for the day or a workout:

- Calves
- Quadriceps
- Hips
- Thoracic spine
- Pectorals

As you may have noticed, the same muscles appear repeatedly throughout this chapter. Despite the number of different sports and injuries, many dysfunctions are interrelated and caused by the same muscles. Many athletes and enthusiasts believe their sport is unique. However, to the human body, all sports involve similar movements. The body should be able to move in specific ranges of motion. If the human body can move and function to its full capacity, you will have reduced your chance of injury—regardless of your activity of choice. Integrate foam rolling into your warm-up as part of a total body dynamic movement prep program. The direct compression of the foam roller onto the muscles will not only improve movement but also improve blood flow to the areas that need it. If you spend just 5 to 10 minutes before a workout to fully prepare the body, you will make a great stride forward on the road to injury prevention.

Chapter 12

FLEXIBILITY

Flexibility is a component of fitness that everyone needs to possess. While you may not need to be as flexible at 80 years old as you did at eight years old, losing the ability to move is associated with increased injuries and decreased quality of life. A large portion of society is negatively affected by flexibility issues.

The National Academy of Sports Medicine defines "flexibility" as the normal extensibility of soft tissue, which allows a joint to be moved through its full motion (McGill & Montel, 2017). In other words, the body should be able to move the way it was designed. A key part of this definition is the use of the words "normal extensibility," because the goal in a flexibility program is to either maintain normal or return to normal.

Too often, individuals seek better than normal; maybe it has something to do with human nature. However, stretching isn't like money: More isn't necessarily better. Only better is better. You can use a specific tool (designed for the joints) to identify what "normal" means to your body. However, you can identify your normal flexibility quicker by performing the assessment in chapter 10. The ability to complete a squat (with acceptable form) usually indicates one is moving well enough to perform the activities they love with minimal chance of injury.

This chapter will begin by discussing the various types of flexibility and how foam rolling can assist in achieving each. Then, it will address common types of stretches. The discussion will explain how to set up and execute each stretch correctly to ensure you are obtaining the most value from the time spent stretching.

TYPES OF FLEXIBILITY TRAINING

As with many aspects of exercise and the human body, there are different types of flexibility training. All of them are effective, but they should be used in a systematic fashion to obtain the most benefit.

Static Stretching

The first type of stretching that can increase flexibility is static stretching. As the name implies, static stretching involves stretching without movement. To do this, you could take muscles to where they feel a small amount of tension and hold for 30 to 45 seconds. The best use of static stretching is usually for adding length to a muscle. While this type of stretching sometimes gets a bad reputation, it is generally just misunderstood. The argument surrounding static stretching is that it reduces force production. This may be true in some situations, but if a muscle has been identified as short and overactive (being too strong in a sense), then a little reduction in force production will do the rest of the body good.

Active Stretching

After you have worked on static stretching for several weeks, you should then progress to active stretching. Here, again as the name implies, the stretch involves some movement. During an active stretch, you could use very similar stretches as in static stretching, but instead of holding for 30 seconds, hold for approximately 2 to 4 seconds. Active stretching is a great way to maintain the flexibility that has been gained from a previous static stretching program and doesn't appear to decrease the force production capabilities of muscle.

Dynamic Stretching

After several weeks of active stretching, move on to common dynamic stretching. Dynamic stretching involves using body weight to take the body through full range of motion exercises. These exercises generally use the same muscle groups as the upcoming workout. Imagine going for a run, for example. A great dynamic warm-up before running may involve performing some leg swings to get the hips moving. In another example, if you are preparing to do an upper body workout, you could perform 10 push-ups. Dynamic stretching is a very popular form of flexibility training before a workout. However, it should only be used after you have regained close to optimal movement. It is very common for individuals to perform dynamic stretches with improper form because they have not taken the time to first work on static and active stretching. Take the time to work through all three types of flexibility over the course of a couple of months.

Foam rolling is indicated for use before all forms of flexibility training. As studies from chapter 1 suggested, foam rolling prior to static stretching has been shown to be the best way to regain normal length in a muscle. In addition, it is frequently recommended that an individual "warm up" prior to stretching. The foam roller helps to increase blood flow to areas of the body that don't receive as much blood flow as muscles, such as tendons and ligaments. In addition, the gentle pressure applied by the foam roller works to reduce tension and alleviate knots that interfere with optimal movement. Therefore, foam rolling serves as an ideal activity to perform before flexibility exercises.

Flexibility exercises usually work best when performed in conjunction with other exercises. For example, you may achieve better results by performing some light strengthening exercises on the muscle opposite the muscle you are stretching. For example, if you have tight quadriceps, follow the flexibility work with light hamstring curls or glute exercises for longer-lasting changes. This works well because these exercises prevent the body from returning to its more comfortable and dysfunctional position. If you have muscle imbalances, the comfortable position is generally one where the tight muscles are allowed to be tight and short—in a position of poor posture. The only way to overcome the tightness, long-term, is to strengthen the muscles.

PROPER STRETCHING TECHNIQUE

To improve flexibility, you must stretch with good form. This is one of the biggest problems I see. Many people think that they can't stretch incorrectly, so they end up getting into all sorts of crazy positions that may be causing more harm than good. You can increase the effectiveness of a stretch simply by paying attention to your posture. The following is a list of muscles that generally need to be stretched, along with the most common postural misalignment and how to fix it. Remember, proper stretching may be uncomfortable, but it shouldn't be painful (unless you're working with a licensed professional who is performing a very specific type of stretching). When going at it alone, avoid further damage by staying aligned and following these simple guidelines—and always foam roll first.

CALVES

The calf muscles are commonly short and problematic for several reasons. The most obvious cause is the footwear we choose to wear. Most individuals wear something with an elevated heel. More and more shoes these days are decreasing the height of the heel, but it is still elevated more than what is natural. The foot is designed to be flat on the ground, with the heel and ball of the foot on the same level. When the heel is elevated, all of the muscles that attach to the bottom of the foot and heel bone and run up the back of the lower leg become short. Over time, these muscles adapt to the shortened position and become tight. This tightness changes how the body moves, which leads to a not-so-obvious cause: calf shortness. When muscles are short, they don't lengthen on cue. So, when walking or running, the body figures out a way to move around the short muscle instead of lengthening it appropriately. This is easy to see if you watch someone walk. Most of the time, people with short calf muscles will turn their toes out significantly further than someone without tight calves. Turning out the toes can exacerbate the tight muscles.

To stretch the calves, begin by standing about an arm's distance from a sturdy wall, and place both hands on the wall. Position the leg to be stretched 6 to 8 inches, or 15.2 to 20.3 centimeters, behind you. Make sure the foot is pointed straight ahead after you reposition it. Then, place the leg that you are not stretching closer to the wall. Contract the quadriceps and glute on the leg to be stretched (see figure 12.1a), and then slowly lean toward the wall (see figure 12.1b). When leaning, move through the ankle joint and not the hip. You should maintain a straight line from the ankle all the way up the body to the ear. Avoid propping your toes up on the wall. While this might give the sensation of improving the stretch in the calves, it stretches the connective tissue on the bottom of the foot. While some people may need to stretch this, most don't. Therefore, for the calf stretch, keep the foot flat on the floor.

If performing static stretching, hold this position for 30 to 45 seconds before switching sides. If performing active stretching, hold for two to four seconds, and then repeat six to eight times before switching sides. If performing dynamic stretching, basic squats or lunges will help the calves and the entire lower body.

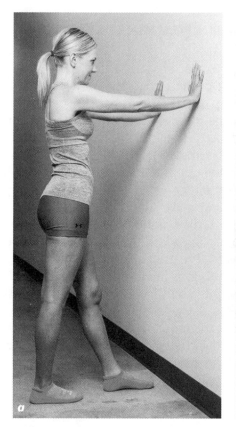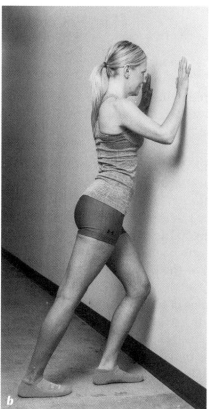

Figure 12.1 Calf stretch.

HIP FLEXORS AND QUADRICEPS

The quadriceps are similar to the calves in that they are large, powerful, and often problematic. Due to the position of these muscles, we are going to stretch the quadriceps along with the hip flexors. There are many great ways to stretch the quadriceps, but one of the most effective ways is to perform the half-kneeling hip flexor and quadriceps stretch.

To stretch the quadriceps and hip flexors, move into a half-kneeling position with one knee down on the floor and the opposite foot on the floor. If you have sensitive knees, place a pad or mat underneath you for comfort. Align your hips over the knee on the floor, and make sure the feet are straight. Next, make sure your pelvis is neutral or turned slightly posterior, which you can do by squeezing the gluteals and tucking a little (see figure 12.2*a*). This is one of the major compensations with this stretch. Far too often people allow the pelvis to dip forward, which shortens the hips flexors and inhibits a stretch. Once in proper position, push the hips forward slowly to the first point of tension (see figure 12.2*b*).

If performing static stretching, hold this position for 30 to 45 seconds before switching sides. If performing active stretching, move slowly through the motion. Then, repeat on the opposite side. Again, for a dynamic stretch of the quadriceps and hip flexors, a basic squat or a squat with rotation works well.

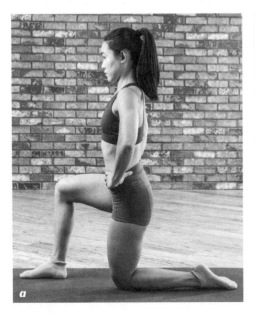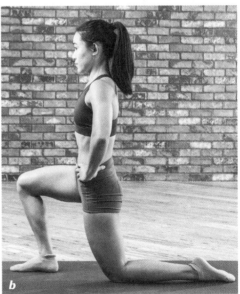

Figure 12.2 Hip flexor and quadriceps stretch.

ADDUCTORS

The adductors are on the inside of the upper leg, but they do more than just bring the legs together. These muscles are positioned in such a way as to assist with everyday movements such as walking or running.

To stretch the adductors, begin in a position with the feet wide (see figure 12.3a). Since each hip can move to about 90 degrees, place the feet significantly further apart than shoulder distance; however, be careful not to put yourself into an unstable position. To best stretch these muscles, keep the feet pointing straight ahead. One of the biggest compensations is to turn the feet outward. While this is not necessarily dangerous, it turns the stretch into more of a hamstring stretch with only a minimal stretch to the adductors. Once in position, keep one leg extended at the knee (this will be the side you're stretching) as you begin to bend the opposite knee (see figure 12.3b). This will shift your weight away from the side you are stretching.

If performing static stretching, take the knee to the first point of tension, hold for 30 to 45 seconds, and then repeat on the other side. If performing active stretching, hold for two to four seconds, and then shift to the other side for two to four seconds. When you progress to dynamic stretching, use a side lunge to prepare the adductors for more strenuous activity.

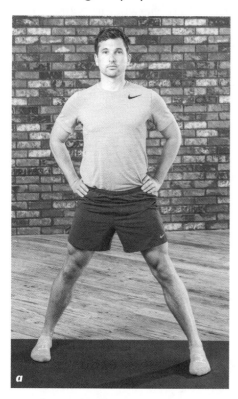 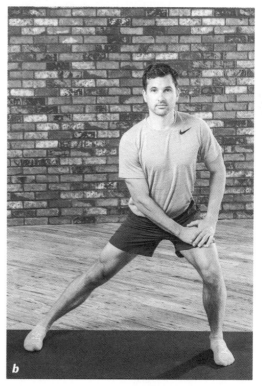

Figure 12.3 Adductors stretch.

HAMSTRINGS

Most people know how to perform at least one type of hamstring stretch. One of the more common ways is to bend down and touch the toes. While this may seem intuitive, it is not as effective as people think. For one, it places stress on the low back. It is also difficult for a muscle to relax if it is working; in a standing position, leaning forward, the hamstrings are definitely working. One of the safest and most effective ways to stretch the hamstrings, if they need it, is by lying flat on your back.

To stretch your hamstrings, lie on a comfortable surface so your spine is neutral (your head should also be flat on the ground). Then, while leaving one leg extended on the ground, bring the other leg up, allowing the knee to bend to a 90-degree angle hip-flexed position (see figure 12.4a). Place both hands around the leg for support, and then use your quadriceps muscle to extend the knee (see figure 12.4b).

Extend until you feel slight discomfort, and hold for 30 to 45 seconds. Not everyone needs to stretch their hamstrings. If you can get your knee fully extended with the hip at a 90-degree angle and don't feel a stretch, then you don't need this one. If performing active stretching, move into the same position and do everything the same way, but only hold for two to four seconds, and perform six to eight repetitions. For a great dynamic hamstring stretch, walk, and perform straight leg kicks. Kick each leg to approximately a 90-degree angle at the hip with the knee extended each time.

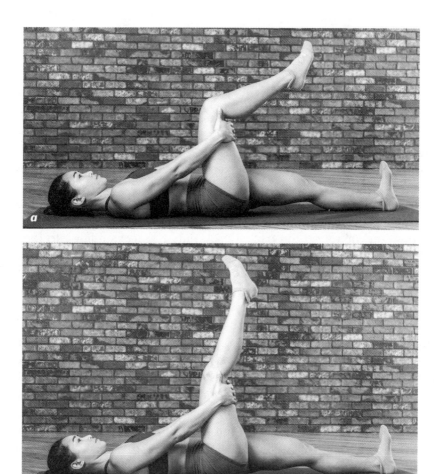

Figure 12.4 Hamstrings stretch.

LATISSIMUS DORSI

The lats extend over a large portion of the back. Therefore, to best stretch this muscle, you will need to consider the position of the arms, back, and pelvis. One of the best stretches I have found for this muscle involves moving into a position that is similar to a child's pose in yoga.

To stretch the lats, kneel on all fours on a comfortable surface with the hands on a roller (see figure 12.5a). Reach both arms all the way out in front of the body, lowering the chest toward the floor (those with really short lats will feel an adequate stretch here), and then slowly lowering your hips back and down to position with your gluteals on your heels (see figure 12.5b). This position will round the back, which puts an ideal stretch into the lats. Hold this position for 30 to 45 seconds. Since you're using both arms at the same time, there is no need to repeat on the other side.

If you have knee or hip problems and can't move into this position, then just perform the exercise for the upper body while standing. Do this by first positioning yourself near a sturdy object with something you can hold. Gym equipment like a weight rack will work. At home, you could grab on to the edge of the sink in the bathroom or kitchen. Then, push your hips back (maybe taking a few steps backward as well) as you bend forward. You will be in the same position as the previous lat stretch, with the arms outstretched, but now you won't be on the ground. If performing active stretching, move into and out of the stretch, holding for two to four seconds and performing six to eight repetitions. A good dynamic stretch for the lats is controlled arm swings. Begin with your hands behind you, and then swing the arms forward and up over your head.

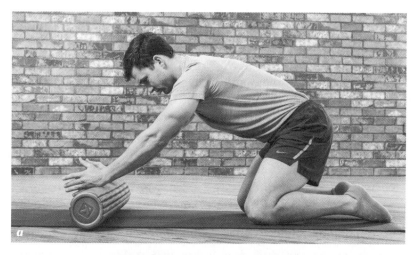

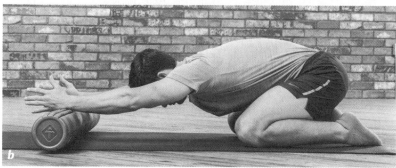

Figure 12.5 Latissimus dorsi stretch.

PECTORALS

The last muscle we will discuss in this section will help the pectoral muscles. These muscles are positioned perfectly to stretch effectively, without requiring you to move into any tricky positions. One of the best ways to stretch the pectorals is to perform a stretch in a doorway.

To stretch the pectorals, begin by standing in an open, single doorway of a normal width. A large, sliding door or French doors are usually too large. Then, place both arms on the outside of the door, with the elbow at approximately shoulder height and bent (see figure 12.6a). Most people with tight chest muscles will already begin to feel this. If you have a little more flexibility, you may want to step one foot forward slightly, so the elbows are now slightly behind the shoulders. Next, squeeze the shoulder blades together to add a little more stretch to the chest (see figure 12.6b). Make sure to keep your head in a neutral position by looking straight ahead. Too often people let the head hang, reducing the effectiveness of the stretch.

Hold this position for 30 to 45 seconds. If performing active stretching, move forward and back holding the stretch for two to four seconds each time. If performing dynamic stretching, basic push-ups will help. If a regular push-up is too challenging, then perform push-ups on a wall or bench to reduce the amount of weight on the arms.

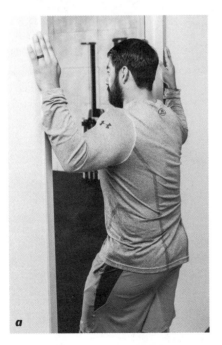 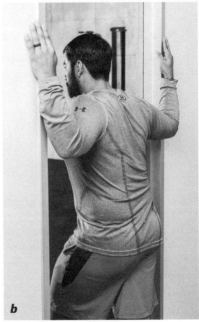

Figure 12.6 Pectorals stretch.

Maintaining ideal flexibility is an important component to health and fitness. Our bodies adapt to the positions we ask them to be in most, even if it's an unhealthy position. Thus, sedentary societies commonly develop muscle imbalances, which lead to aches, pains, and injuries. The foam roller can be used to assist in flexibility training, but foam rolling alone is not the most effective routine. Use foam rolling in conjunction with other techniques and strengthening exercises for longer-lasting results.

Chapter 13

RECOVERY

Recovery is one of the most popular uses of the foam roller. This was definitely supported in the research discussed in chapter 1. This book has described many effective uses of foam rolling, such as preparation and during a workout. It is also an incredibly effective method of recovery. This chapter will discuss some of the reasons why it works so well for recovery and detail some foam rolling techniques that may be better suited for recovery.

HOW FOAM ROLLING BENEFITS RECOVERY

The first thing to consider is what issue you are trying to recover from. Usually, "recovery" is used to mean the period of time after a workout, athletic activity, or any sort of exercise. While true, this is not the only time we need to recover. Any time the body is stressed—physically, psychologically, or even emotionally—you may need some sort of recovery. Take the workplace, for example. If you sit in a chair at an office like I do for several hours a day, most days of the week, you are stressing the body. A lack of movement can lead to just as many injuries as moving too much. In fact, these injuries are often classified the same: repetitive strain injuries or overuse injuries. Remember, foam rolling not only increases blood and fluid flow but also moves tissues around. This essentially "unsticks" areas of the body that are stuck from a lack of use. Therefore, foam rolling after a long day of sitting would also serve as an effective recovery.

There are two common areas the average, sedentary office worker complains about most: the lower back and the upper back or neck. (I address the upper back and neck here as one area, as addressing one usually helps both.)

The root causes of discomfort in these areas have been discussed in previous chapters, but these two conditions can benefit greatly from just a few minutes on the foam roller for the simple reason that rolling introduces movement to painful areas. This reason alone should motivate you to use the foam roller periodically throughout the day. Rolling throughout the day helps to decrease the severity of discomfort at the end of the day. The body is sensitive to time. A small amount of stress is not bad—in fact, it is beneficial. However, a small amount of stress applied to the body for days, weeks, and months can wreak havoc. I have often heard the analogy of the small stream of water that, as it flows, produces the Grand Canyon over a period of millions of years. If you can reduce stress throughout the day or, at a minimum, at the end of the day by introducing a little foam rolling into your daily routine, you can help prevent a big injury, ache, or pain in the future.

The foam roller can also assist with recovery after a workout, with a few added key components. During a workout, muscles and connective tissue are damaged. The damage is not severe in most cases, which means the body will recover without any problems. A condition called rhabdomyolysis (commonly called "rhabdo") involves damage that is too extensive or has occurred too quickly. Although relatively rare, due to a recent trend in exercise that is incredibly intense, this condition is occurring more frequently. Working out can cause small tears in muscle fibers. When there is little damage, the body repairs the muscle, making it bigger and stronger. Rhabdo occurs when the muscle damage is so bad that the contents of the muscle fiber are released into the blood stream. Too much of this release can cause problems. If you suffer from rhabdo during a workout, it means you did not properly plan your workout. Exercise should never be so intense that enough muscle damage occurs to essentially poison you. Foam rolling will likely have little to no benefit in cases of rhabdo.

During normal or even intense exercise, microtears cause some pain and discomfort as the body repairs itself. The pain comes from a small amount of inflammation that accompanies the damage, but this is actually beneficial. Inflammation is often seen in a negative light. However, it's an important part of recovery for the body. Swelling or inflammation occurs when the body sends extra nutrients to the damaged tissue, thus repairing it.

In the strength and conditioning industry, there is frequent discussion around anti-inflammatory medication and its role in muscle growth. While the research is limited, it appears that taking an anti-inflammatory after a workout designed to increase muscle size will have negative effects on muscle growth (Trappe et al., 2002). The bottom line is that inflammation is valuable. However, too much inflammation or inflammation that lasts too long can also have negative consequences (discussed in more detail in chapter 14). Therefore, one way to allow the body to repair itself naturally, while preventing an accumulation of inflammatory fluid, is to increase blood flow around the tissues. You can do this by using a foam roller after a workout to assist in flushing out the old blood and bringing in new blood.

When using the foam roller as a recovery tool, the same rules can apply. First, slowly roll the muscle, about 1 inch, or 2.5 centimeters, per second to identify tender spots. When a spot is found, hold pressure for about 30 seconds or until the tenderness begins to reduce. This is an especially valuable method to use on the muscles identified as overactive or short in your movement assessment. These muscles are prone to becoming short, likely due to repetitive patterns and adaptation, so addressing them again in the cool-down is recommended. In fact, rolling them the exact same way and re-stretching them would be ideal. These muscles could use this treatment several times per day. However, there is another aspect to consider when using the foam roller for recovery that focuses specifically on the increases in blood and fluid flow throughout the musculature.

When muscles work hard, they use energy. This energy comes in the form of a molecule called adenosine triphosphate (ATP). In order to produce energy, ATP breaks a bond, which produces an energy by-product. (I generally refer to this as "metabolic waste."). The body is well equipped to clean out this metabolic waste, as long as it isn't accumulating too quickly. At lower levels of intensity with close-to-regular rates of breathing, the consistent blood flow and oxygen cleans out this waste.

When this happens, the muscles feel good and work well. However, at high rates of energy production, the metabolic waste begins to build up. There simply isn't enough blood and oxygen flowing to get it all out, so it begins to accumulate. This is usually felt as a burning sensation in the muscles. However, this is not lactic acid, as has been taught over the years. It is hydrogen that is affecting the pH levels of the body (pH stands for percent of hydrogen). This happens more in the muscles that are doing most of the work for a particular exercise or movement. It is well known that a light cool-down after a workout will help to flush out the body and assist in recovery. However, we also know now that several of these molecules are very large and must be pushed out. This means that a light walk may not be as beneficial as everyone once thought. (It should be noted that walking as a cool-down is never a bad idea and has no negative consequence, but there could be a better option.)

A better option in this situation would be to apply pressure directly to the muscles that were working the hardest during the workout or activity. The pressure will encourage the large molecules to move into the blood stream better, allowing fresh blood and oxygen to come in and begin the repair process. In these cases, there does not appear to be a wrong way to foam roll. Any movement will get everything flowing better than doing nothing. However, I have found that maintaining a slow but steady rolling pace is most beneficial. In addition, I recommend a slightly softer foam roller for these recovery sessions. The goal here is not necessarily to induce pain, or really even to find tender spots, but to push out metabolic waste and allow fresh nutrients to take its place.

To roll specifically for recovery—keeping in mind this may not relieve tightness or improve muscle imbalances but will push nutrients around—begin with a softer roller at the calves and slowly work your way up. What follows is approximately a 10-minute program that can be used for recovery from a workout. This will be a total body recovery routine, so think about doing this after a total body workout. However, if you are focusing on the lower body for your workout, then you can direct your foam rolling to the lower body. The goal of our recovery rolling is not to work as deep as possible, but there may still be considerable discomfort. The goal, as has been mentioned several times, is nutrient flow. Therefore, on each of the body parts below, you may choose how much pressure you would like. In many cases, for areas such as the lower body, you can place both legs on the roller at the same time for just the right amount of pressure and to take up less time. While you can cross one leg over the other for increased pressure, this is not a requirement. The programming for each of the following is simple: Roll at a slow and consistent pace, from the bottom of the muscle to the top. Hold if you would like, but again, it isn't required. Whatever you do, don't roll quickly. Fast rolling generates friction but doesn't actually move fluid as well as slow rolling.

FOAM ROLLING TECHNIQUES FOR RECOVERY

Any muscle in the body may be rolled using recovery techniques, although I have found that the muscle groups listed here appear to benefit the most from recovery rolling.

Lower Body Recovery

Lower body recovery rolling includes more areas than the upper body, due to the nature of our lower body musculature. We have more muscles in the lower body that are large and powerful so we can efficiently move our upper body from point A to point B. Since these muscles are larger, you may have to reposition yourself slightly as you roll. There is no right or wrong way to reposition, but try to maintain good posture, roll slowly, and breathe throughout each technique.

CALVES

Begin by placing the foam roller just above the ankle. Cross one leg over the other for more pressure, or roll both at the same time (for the body position when rolling one leg, see figure 13.1*a*). Place your hands near your hips. Raise your hips just off the ground, and then push yourself forward so the roller comes up toward the back of your knee (see figure 13.1*b*). Try to roll from the ankle to the knee in one motion if possible. Then, return by letting the hips come back and allowing the roller to move back to the ankle. Repeat this 4 to 5 times or approximately 60 seconds at a slow pace. If rolling with the legs crossed, switch legs to repeat the rolling.

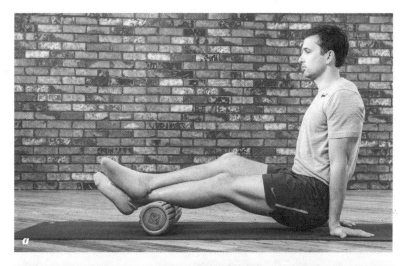

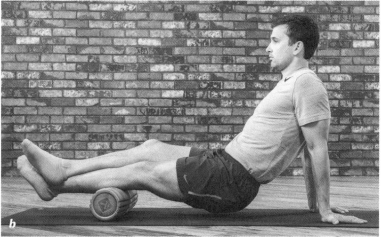

Figure 13.1   Foam rolling the calf for recovery.

QUADRICEPS

Begin by placing the foam roller just above the knee. Both legs may be placed on the roller or you may roll one leg at a time (for the body position when rolling one leg at a time, see figure 13.2a). Place the elbows under the shoulders. Ideally, the leg would be rolled in one smooth motion from knee to hip. In order to do this, the elbows will likely have to move during the rolling. When ready, push your body down, so the foam roller comes up toward the hips (see figure 13.2b). Don't overextend your back to move the roller all the way up—just step the elbows down one to two times. Then pull your body back up so that the roller moves toward the knee, again stepping the elbows up as necessary until the roller is near the knees again. Repeat this 4 to 5 times or for approximately 60 seconds at a slow pace.

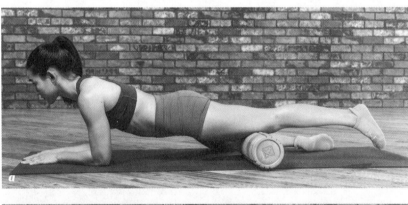

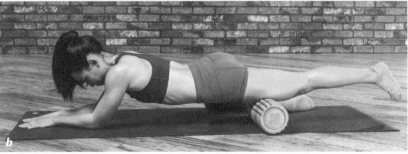

Figure 13.2 Foam rolling the quadriceps for recovery.

IT Band

First, remember that when we say iliotibial (IT) band, we actually mean that large muscle of the quadriceps under the IT band: the vastus lateralis. Since this area is very tender in most people and requires an awkward position, I recommend you use two foam rollers at the same time if you have them. It will be far more tolerable (and thus effective) for this type of rolling. If you have only one roller, place the roller just below the hip joint and perpendicular to the thigh (see figure 13.3*a*). If you use two rollers, you will notice that it is less painful than using one roller because you are displacing your body weight across two rollers. The elbow should be below the shoulder with the opposite hand and foot placed in front of the body for support. Again, ideally, to flush out metabolic waste from this muscle, the entire area would be rolled slowly. If using two rollers at the same time, you will notice you don't need to reposition the elbow much, if at all. Begin by pushing yourself down so the roller comes up the leg to bottom of the hip (see figure 13.3*b*), and then roll the other direction. Repeat this 4 to 5 times or approximately 60 seconds at a slow pace. You cannot roll both legs at the same time, so repeat the entire process on the other leg before moving on.

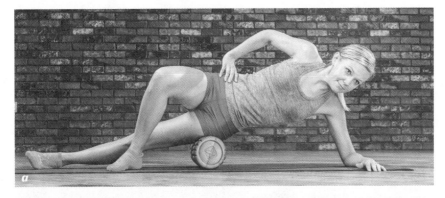

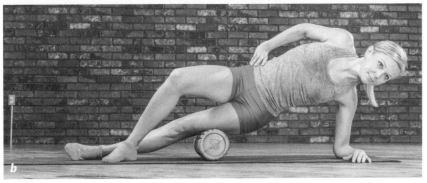

Figure 13.3　Foam rolling the IT band for recovery.

Hamstrings

The hamstrings should never be the hardest-working muscle in an activity. Many people like to isolate the hamstrings, but in total body lifts, such as squats, deadlifts, and lunges (which are always more effective), the hamstrings are a mere helper. If your hamstrings are much sorer than the gluteals or quadriceps after "leg day," then you probably have a hamstring issue, as the hamstrings are being asked to do much more than they should. However, given the many problems that occur in the hamstrings (discussed in previous chapters), I don't think it is bad to roll them after lower body work. This offers an opportunity to get things flowing. However, rolling the hamstrings for recovery should rarely take priority over the quadriceps. These are different types of muscles with different goals. Begin by placing the foam roller just above the knee on the back of the leg. Both legs may be placed on the roller or you may roll one leg at a time (for the body position when rolling both legs at the same time, see figure 13.4a). Place the hands near your hips. Raise your hips and slowly push your body down so the roller comes up the back of the legs toward the hips (see figure 13.4b). Try to move the roller all the way up to the hips in one smooth motion, repositioning the hands if necessary. Then, pull the body up so the roller travels down toward the knees. Repeat this 4 to 5 times or approximately 60 seconds at a slow pace.

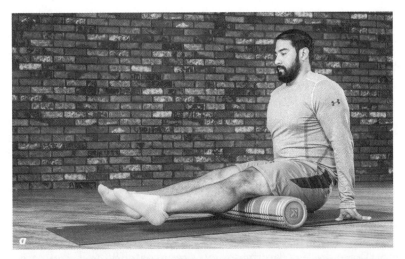

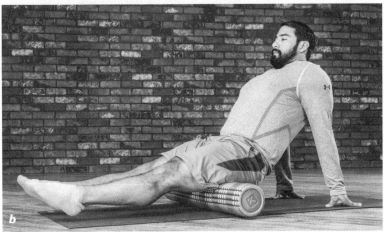

Figure 13.4 Foam rolling the hamstrings for recovery.

GLUTEALS

Optimally functioning gluteals should be working very hard in almost every workout, especially workouts targeting the lower body. However, I usually hear about sore quadriceps and hamstrings, as the glutes don't work to their full capacity in many people. Remember, the rolling routine in this chapter is specific to recovery and does not integrate the same techniques used in preparation. If you think your glutes should be doing more work, refer back to the assessment in chapter 10. The glutes are difficult to roll at the same time. I suggest you focus on one glute at a time by shifting your weight onto one hip. There is little need to cross one leg over the other. Crossing the leg while rolling the glute can help to target smaller muscles in the hip. However, our intent for recovery is not so much to release the muscle as it is to encourage recovery. Therefore, I recommend you simply extend the leg you are rolling so it is relaxed on the ground. Sit directly on top of the foam roller, allowing the leg to be rolled to relax out in front (see figure 13.5a). Place one arm on the ground near the hip so your body is leaning back slightly on the roller. Begin rolling by pushing the body down so the roller comes up toward the low back. You do not need to make a large rolling motion. Then, pull your body back up so the roller moves toward the leg (see figure 13.5b). Again, due to the size of the roller, you only need to roll a couple of inches, or a few centimeters, up and down. Repeat this 4 to 5 times or approximately 60 seconds at a slow pace. You can't roll both legs at the same time, so repeat the entire process on the other leg before moving on.

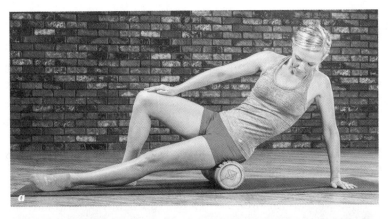

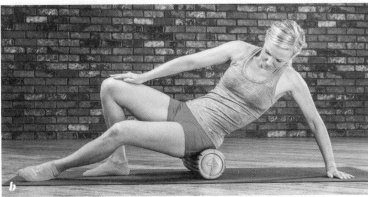

Figure 13.5 Foam rolling the glutes for recovery.

Upper Body Recovery

Upper body recovery is not as extensive as the lower body—not because it's not important, but because the muscles doing the most work in the upper body (the latissimus dorsi and pectorals) are tough to target. The lats, for example, span a large portion of the torso and areas, such as the lower back, that shouldn't be foam rolled frequently. The pectorals attach to the arm and travel toward the torso, attaching to the clavicle, sternum, and ribs. With the presence of breast tissue and mammary ducts in both men and women, it is painful and potentially dangerous to roll across the entire chest. Therefore, only small portions of these muscles can be safely rolled.

LATISSIMUS DORSI

The latissimus dorsi (lats) contributes to many motions of the shoulder. Therefore, the lats can become very sore after upper body workouts. Only a small portion of the lats can be safely rolled. Begin by placing the roller just below one shoulder blade, with the body lying on one side (see figure 13.6a). The arm on the side to be rolled must be relaxed, so it is often best to let it simply lie on the floor. The arm you are not rolling may be used for support. Raise the hips off the ground with the legs, and use the legs to pull the body down so the roller moves toward the armpit (see figure 13.6b). Roll down far enough for the roller to get to the armpit and almost to the arm. Then, use the lower body and opposite arm to push the body back up so the roller moves back to the bottom of the shoulder blade. Repeat this 4 to 5 times or approximately 60 seconds at a slow pace. Repeat the entire process on the other lat before moving on.

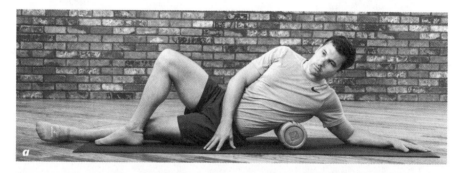

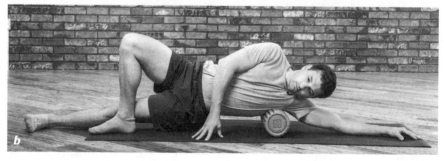

Figure 13.6 Foam rolling the lats for recovery.

PECTORALS

The pectorals are large muscles that can do a lot of work. Many people focus a significant amount of time developing their pecs. If people just stood with better posture, their pectorals would immediately appear more defined. At any rate, the pectorals can feel very sore and warrant the use of some foam rolling recovery. As mentioned previously, although the pectorals cover a good deal of the upper torso, due to breast tissue and other sensitivities, it is not a great idea to try to roll the entire muscle. Therefore, focus on the more lateral portion. Lie face down with the roller positioned under the shoulder on the pec you wish to address first. The arm on the side being rolled should be relaxed. Use the opposite arm to slightly lift that side (see figure 13.7a). Push the body toward the roller so the roller moves toward the midline of the body (see figure 13.7b). Then, pull the body with the arm so the roller moves back toward the shoulder. Repeat this 4 to 5 times or for approximately 60 seconds at a slow pace. Repeat the entire process on the other pec before moving on.

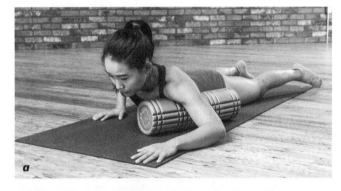

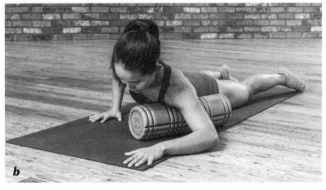

Figure 13.7 Foam rolling the pectorals for recovery.

I need to reiterate one last time that this type of rolling is specific to recovery and should be used as such. Rolling in this fashion is intended to flush out metabolic waste from muscles that have been working the hardest, allowing fresh blood and oxygen to take its place, thereby speeding up recovery. If you are dealing with aches, pains, muscle imbalances, or injuries, this type of rolling is not harmful, but it may not be the best for you. If you have any questions about whether you should complete this rolling routine, refer back to chapter 10 and complete the assessment. Use the rolling techniques in section 2 on the muscles identified as overactive and short or tight. The recovery techniques in this chapter are designed for people who move relatively well and are training with higher-intensity workouts. The high intensity is what leads to the waste accumulation and potential soreness. That type of training warrants the use of this type of foam rolling.

Chapter 14

REHABILITATION

The general public often overlooks the importance of restoring normal function after injury. If you don't spend time rehabilitating after an injury, you greatly increase the chance of additional injuries. In fact, one of the biggest predictors of a future injury is a past injury. Paterno and colleagues found that sustaining one knee injury that requires surgery increases the chance of another knee injury by 25 percent (2012). However, the second injury often doesn't happen to the same knee. The opposite knee becomes more at risk of injury. Also, this does not mean that the second injury will be the same type of injury at all. It is common to see someone first experience an ankle sprain, or something nonthreatening, but rush the rehabilitation and then end up experiencing a debilitating hamstring tear. Many sports medicine doctors and athletic trainers recognize this and make sure to completely rehabilitate the first injury before allowing a high-profile athlete back on the court or field. This same level of service should be given to all individuals when they experience injuries. While an ankle sprain may not mean you need to call in sick at work, if you are an avid runner, then your physical activities should be limited until your function has fully returned. This chapter will introduce and explore the complicated process of an injury (frequently referred to as "the cumulative injury cycle") including a brief description of corrective exercises.

THE CUMULATIVE INJURY CYCLE

The problem with attempting to do too much too soon can be traced to our natural ability to adapt to less-than-ideal circumstances. When your ankle is sprained, it is natural to avoid using it. Therefore, you limp. A limp may allow you to travel from point A to point B, but if the ankle is sprained, you cannot move optimally. Limping increases the amount of calories you expend to complete movements and increases stresses in nearby joints, such as the knee or hip. If this occurs for too long, limping becomes normal and you may continue favoring that one injury. Before you know it, you're suffering from low back pain that you can't explain. That doesn't mean you must go on bed rest after a minor injury. In fact, the opposite is true in most cases. You often need to use the injured body part in order to rehabilitate. This is where the phrase "walk it off" comes from. After an ankle sprain, for example, moving it encourages blood flow, reduces inflammation, and may lead to quicker recovery. However, moving the ankle does not mean performing repetitive box jumps or continuing your marathon training. Common sense can take you a long way with rehabilitation. Use an injured joint only up to where the pain begins, and, more importantly, give it time to rest.

Injuries generally follow the cumulative injury cycle, a cycle that could be vicious if it reinforces itself over time. This is how minor injuries turn into big problems or how failing to take proper care of an injury leads to another injury. Additionally, this cycle provides insight into how and when foam rolling should take place as it relates to an injury. The cumulative injury cycle encompasses six steps:

1. *Tissue trauma:* This is the result of the injury. It is the initial damage to the muscle or connective tissue.

2. *Inflammation:* The normal response to most injuries or tissue damage is swelling or inflammation around the traumatized area. The swelling brings specialized cells to the injury to begin the repair process and also initiates a pain response. This happens in an attempt to reduce more damage. When something hurts, you are much less likely to use it.

3. *Muscle spasm:* This works along with inflammation but may last longer. When an area of the body is injured, the muscles around it will often tighten to protect the joint. This prevents painful movement that may lead to more injury.

4. *Adhesions:* As previous chapters mentioned, if muscles and other tissues aren't able to slide freely across one another, then the body begins to lay down additional tissue and develops knots or adhesions (basically an internal scar). This leads to tightness, which reduces flexibility and the ability to fully use the muscle.

5. *Altered nervous and muscular system control:* When the adhesions prevent normal movement, then the body must learn how to coordinate movement in a different way. As previously discussed, if one muscle is tight and inflexible, then another muscle is lengthened and unable to do its job completely. This changes movement patterns over time and applies more stress to one area while another area loses adequate stress.

6. *Development of muscle imbalance:* As the body alters its nervous and muscular system control day after day, the pattern is reinforced and a muscle imbalance develops. Muscle imbalances change large movement patterns, allowing other parts of the body to now be more susceptible to injury. This is how an individual may be at increased risk of a shoulder injury due to an ankle sprain a few years earlier.

Foam rolling can play a part in interfering with muscle spasms and adhesions. In a more serious injury, you may need to let the body have its muscle spasms, thereby preventing more injury. Then, you could use the foam roller to help break up and mobilize the adhesions that are almost sure to develop. In a less serious injury, where the muscle spasm may be working as a faulty protection system, the foam roller could be used on the muscle that is spasming. Theoretically, this may prevent the adhesions from ever occurring—and if the adhesions don't show up, then neither will steps 5 and 6. In this case, the cycle is broken or will not repeat itself.

Of course the decision about when to begin foam rolling will depend on the type and severity of injury. To simplify this discussion, I prefer to categorize injuries into (1) major injuries (those that require help from a clinician) and (2) minor injuries (those that do not require help from a clinician). It is up to you to decide which type of injury you have. If you experienced an injury accompanied by a loud popping noise, followed by significant bruising; if there is an open wound; if you think a bone is broken; or if you are sure something is terribly wrong, consult a physician. That is something that should be assessed as soon as possible, and sticking a foam roller in there may do more harm than good.

I will classify a minor injury as a basic sprain, an injury with minimal to no bruising or some swelling, or any injury that you can sort of "walk off," albeit with a little pain. Major injuries, those resulting in significant bruising, swelling, and usually accompanied by a loud pop, may be complete muscle or ligament tears (off the bone or in half). These generally require surgery and extensive rehabilitation with a physical therapist. However, many minor sprains or strains do not require a major intervention, such as a surgery, but may benefit from the help of a physical therapist. The therapist will be able to assess the damaged tissue, provide treatment, and create a follow-up plan to be completed at home. The foam roller will likely be a part of all take-home plans. Professor Shirley Sahrmann was well known for the importance she placed on self-care plans. She stated that most of the benefits of therapy were achieved at home and the purpose of seeing the therapist was to reassess and ensure that the patient was executing exercises correctly (2002).

After an injury, when tissue is healing, it lays down additional tissue in a random pattern. Imagine how a piece of canvas would look if you threw an entire gallon of paint at it—it would just be a big splotch. Much like the paint on the canvas, we can influence how scar tissue develops by frequently moving the body. If you've had a deep cut or surgery, you're probably familiar with how a scar feels close to the surface. It may be thick, and you can feel a denseness to the tissue in that area. The same thing happens down in the muscle, except thickness that deep in the muscles could lead to more pain and injury. Scar tissue is inelastic: It doesn't stretch easily, and if it does, it doesn't return to its original length. We need to use the foam roller and exercises to interfere or prevent this as much as possible.

To achieve the best results, you will need to integrate foam rolling with additional exercises. They are not difficult or challenging exercises but do include movement. The goal is to use the foam roller to break up knots or adhesions, and then use movement in various stages to encourage develop-ment of additional scar tissue. This action works based on a principle known as Davis's Law, which states that soft tissue will lay down along the lines of stress. The stress induced by proper movement means the scar will be what I call a "functional scar." Functional scars allow movement to occur naturally, without restriction. We can't stop scar tissue from developing—nor would we want to—but we can prevent them from becoming "dysfunctional." Dysfunc-tional scars limit movement, increase the chance of another injury, and often cause pain. In order to increase the chance of turning scars into functional tissue, you will first want to foam roll, then stretch and complete a few simple exercises. Performing specific exercises after increasing flexibility helps to better retain the changes made.

CORRECTIVE EXERCISE PROGRAMS

To truly rehabilitate after an injury, you must prepare yourself to return to optimal function (the ability to do whatever you'd like to do when you'd like to do it). Far too often I see people who are unable to return to the activities they love after what should be an insignificant injury. This usually occurs because the individual either doesn't know there is a process or chooses the wrong process. I recommend the corrective exercise program suggested by the National Academy of Sports Medicine. It is thorough yet simple and very effective. Corrective exercise should not be confused with rehab. Rehab is a term reserved for a clinician, whereas anyone can do corrective exercise. Corrective exercise is intended to occur after rehabilitation for more serious injuries and to ensure people return optimal function. However, corrective exercise can also be used for minor injuries or, ideally, used on a daily basis to prevent injuries. Therefore, corrective exercise targets the body as a whole and does not focus solely on one particular injury.

Corrective exercise programs begin by identifying the area of the body that needs to be addressed. As covered in chapter 10, the most effective way to do this is to perform an assessment. If you skipped the chapter or need a refresher, take a few minutes to glance at it. The assessment will direct you to the area that needs the most work. This is important because many times this is not where the injury occurred. Take, for example, an ankle sprain. Certainly some muscles around the ankle play a role in the sprain, but muscles at the hips also affect the ankle. Thus, foam rolling, stretching, and strengthening the areas of the ankle may only achieve minimal results if the hips are the problem. From the perspective of mobility or a tight muscle, the assessment generally identifies short and restricted muscles in the calves and hips and in the upper body around the chest muscles and the lats. The assessment also usually identifies weaknesses in the muscles in the feet, some hip muscles, and in the upper back. Once you have this information, you can begin a corrective exercise program.

Use the programs that follow as a guide to accompany your assessment. These routines offer a great place to begin and will help you achieve great results. This is not an exhaustive list but suggests a few areas to work on once a day, five days a week, for about three to four weeks. If you are seeing the results you desire, stick with it. If you don't begin seeing results within about three weeks, revisit your assessment to check that you're targeting the correct areas. Each program will consist of four parts: (1) foam rolling, (2) performing one to two stretches, (3) simple exercises intended to emphasize specific muscles, and (4) a total body exercise. The total body movement will assist in relearning a movement pattern. All four steps are imperative—first to add length to short, problematic muscles and second to reteach the body how to move.

Researchers Grooms, Appelbaum, and Onate found that after a knee injury, the brain has to relearn the ideal movement pattern (2015). This is true for all injuries, so think of this as a learning experience for the body.

FEET TURN OUT

If the feet turn out, it may be associated with feet, knee, and hip pain or ankle sprains. The following is recommended:

- *Foam roll*: Bottom of the feet and the calves
- *Stretch*: Standing calf stretch
- *Isolated exercise*: Towel scrunches and specialized calf raises
- *Total body exercise*: Single leg balance with variations of movement when necessary

KNEES MOVE IN

If the knees move in, it may be associated with feet or hip pain or ankle sprains. This is highly associated with knee injuries during activity. The following is recommended:

- *Foam roll*: Calves, quadriceps, and adductors
- *Stretch*: Standing calf stretch, standing adductor stretch, and half-kneeling quadriceps stretch
- *Isolated exercise*: Side-lying leg raise up against a wall
- *Total body exercise*: Assisted squat with tubing around knees

EXCESSIVE FORWARD LEAN

Excessive forward lean is frequently linked to low back pain and may be associated with ankle sprains. The following is recommended:

- *Foam roll*: Calves and TFL
- *Stretch*: Standing calf stretch and half-kneeling quadriceps stretch
- *Isolated exercise*: Heel walks and opposite arm and leg raise (bird dog)
- *Total body exercise*: Front squat or squat with cables or tubing attached near the ground

ANTERIOR PELVIC TILT

Anterior pelvic tilt is closely associated with low back pain and is also an indicator of weak core muscles (which has been linked to many injuries including ankle sprains and knee and shoulder injuries). The following is recommended:

- *Foam roll*: Quadriceps, TFL, piriformis, and lats
- *Stretch*: Half-kneeling quadriceps stretch and child's pose lat stretch with foam roller
- *Isolated exercise*: Glute bridge and plank or dead bug
- *Total body exercise*: Ball wall or assisted squat

ARMS FALL FORWARD

Arms that fall forward are associated with shoulder injuries, neck pain, and upper back tightness. The following is recommended:

- *Foam roll*: Thoracic spine, pecs, and lats
- *Stretch*: Thoracic spine stretch with foam roller and child's pose lat stretch with foam roller
- *Isolated exercise*: Shoulder retractions and depression (cobra) and stability ball and standing shoulder raises, or scaption raises; these should be performed with the thumbs pointing up and with the arms about 45 degrees in front of the body
- *Total body exercise*: Standing wide grip high row with tubing or cables

To reiterate, the programs here are simple and to the point. If you have not suffered an injury, then use the above programs as part of your warm-up before exercising or before participating in an athletic event. Once you learn your routine, it should not take longer than 10 minutes to complete. This will provide a superior way to prepare for activities than the often-used warm-up on a treadmill. In addition, these movements will target muscles specific to your movement patterns, preparing your body for the increased stress to come. Keep in mind, this may not be ideal if you have recently suffered a major injury. These programs can be used after you have been released from physical therapy or may be used if dealing with a minor injury. Be aware of form and posture during the exercises listed in this chapter. Always concentrate on keeping the spine neutral and moving slowly, trying to feel each movement. For my clients, I request that they not listen to music during this time or, if they do, that they listen to something soft and slow. This encourages them to concentrate on what they are doing. It's like learning a new language or really learning anything new—you need concentration and "deep practice," as author Daniel Coyle (*The Talent Code*) calls it. Deep practice means focusing your attention on exactly what you're doing. If you make a mistake, immediately go back and fix it, making sure to never repeat or reinforce the mistakes. You will find that this is not easy. The body wants to cheat by compensating and taking the easy route. That route is usually paved with more injuries, frustration, and failure in exercise programs.

Foam rolling is a great addition to a program to help boost performance by improving movement patterns, increasing blood flow, speeding up recovery, and helping reduce pain. These benefits can be achieved if foam rolling is used every day or even just most days of the week. This book has covered everything you need to know about getting started with foam rolling: beginning with the science of foam rolling, progressing to the history and safety, and finally implementing a successful foam rolling programming. However you choose to integrate foam rolling into your day to get the best results, base what you roll on how you move. If you're unsure of how you move, chapter 10 walks you through a simple assessment. If this presents too many challenges, then refer to chapter 11 for some basic rolling programs. Last, but not least, add motions in addition to just rolling. Perform a few side-to-side motions along with some pin-and-stretch movements to make sure you're making the most of your time on the roller. Thanks for rolling with me.

REFERENCES

Chapter 1

Barnes, M.F. (1997). The basic science of myofascial release: Morphologic change in connective tissue. *Journal of Bodywork and Movement Therapies, 1*(4), 231-239.

Chan, Y., Wang, T., Chang, C., Chen, L., Chu, H., Lin, S., & Chang, S. (2015). Short-term effects of self-massage combined with home exercise on pain, daily activity, and autonomic function in patients with myofascial pain dysfunction syndrome. *Journal of Physical Therapy Science, 27,* 217-225.

Cheatham, S.W., Kolber, M.J., Cain, M., & Lee, M. (2015). The effects of self-myofascial release using a foam roll or roller massager on joint range of motion, muscle recovery, and performance: A systematic review. *The International Journal of Sports Physical Therapy, 10*(6), 827-838.

Clark, M.A. (2000). *Integrated training for the new millennium.* Thousand Oaks, CA: National Academy of Sports Medicine.

Clark, M.A., & Lucett, S.C. (2011). *NASM essentials of corrective exercise training.* Philadelphia, PA: Lippincott Williams & Wilkins.

Delaney, J.P., Leong, K.S., Watkins, A., & Brodie, D. (2002). The short-term effects of myofascial trigger point massage therapy on cardiac autonomic tone in health subjects. *Journal of Advanced Nursing, 37*(4), 364-371.

Edmunds, R., Dettelbach, A., Dito, J., Kirkpatrick, A., Parra, A., Souder, J. . . . Astorino, T.A. (2016). Effects of foam rolling versus static stretching on recovery of quadriceps and hamstrings force. *Journal of Bodywork and Movement Therapies, 20* (1), 146.

Fleisher, T., Griffin, L., Jensen, J., Pratt, S., & Gupta, D. (2013). The acute effects of two different self-myofascial release products on calf muscle pump and ankle range of motion. Poster presented at American Physical Therapy Association: Combined Sections Meeting, Indianapolis, IN.

Healey, K.C., Hatfield, D.L., Blanpied, P., Dorfman, L.R., & Riebe, D. (2013). The effects of myofascial release with foam rolling on performance. *Journal of Strength and Conditioning Research, 28*(1), 61-68.

Kim, K., Park, S., Goo, B., & Choi, S. (2014). Effect of self-myofascial release on reduction of physical stress: A pilot study. *Journal of Physical Therapy Science, 26,* 1779-1781.

Lanigan, C.S., & Harrison, A.J. (2012). The effects of self myofascial release on the plantar surface of the foot during single leg rebound jumps. *Journal of Bodywork and Movement Therapies. [Abstract].*

MacDonald, G.Z., Button, D.C., Drinkwater, E.J., & Behm, D.G. (2014). Foam rolling as a recovery tool after an intense bout of physical activity. *Medicine & Science in Sports & Exercise, 46(1),* 131-142.

Markovic, G. (2015). Acute effects of instrument assisted soft tissue mobilization vs. foam rolling on knee and hip range of motion in soccer players. *Journal of Bodywork and Movement Therapies, 19,* 690-696.

Okamoto, T., Masuhara, M., & Ikuta, K. (2014). Acute effects of self-myofascial release using a foam roller on arterial function. *Journal of Strength and Conditioning Research, 28*(1), 69-73.

Peacock, C.A., Krein, D.D., Silver, T.A., Sanders, G.J., & Von Carlowitz, K.P.A. (2014). An acute bout of self-myofascial release in the form of foam rolling improves performance testing. *International Journal of Exercise Science, 7*(3), 202-2011.

Pearcy, G.E., Bradbury-Squires, D.J., Kawamoto, J.E., Drinkwater, E.J., Behm, D.G., & Button, D.C. (2015). Foam rolling for delayed-onset muscle soreness and recovery of dynamic performance measures. *Journal of Athletic Training, 50*(1), 5-13.

Schroeder, A.N., & Best, T.M. (2015). Is self myofascial release an effective preexercise and recovery strategy? A literature review. *Current Sports Medicine Reports (ACSM), 14*(3), 200-208.

Skarabot, J., Beardsley, C., & Stirn, I. (2015). Comparing the effects of self-myofascial release with static stretching on ankle range-of-motion in adolescent athletes. *International Journal of Sports Physical Therapy, 10*(2), 203-212.

Sullivan, K.M., Silvey, D.B., Button, D.C., & Behm, D.G. (2013). Roller-massager application to the hamstrings increases sit-and-reach range of motion within five to ten seconds without performance impairments. *The International Journal of Sports Physical Therapy, 8*(3), 228-236.

Takamoto, K., Sakai, S., Hori, E., Urakawa, S., Umeno, K., Ono, T., & Nishijo, H. (2009). Compression on trigger points in the leg muscle increases parasympathetic nervous activity based on heart rate variability. *Journal of Physiological Sciences, 59*(3), 191-197.

Travell, J., Simons, D., & Simons, L. (1999). *Myofascial pain and dysfunction: The trigger point manual* (2nd ed., Volume 1). Philadelphia, PA: Lippincott Williams & Wilkins.

Chapter 2

Butler, D., & Moseley, L. (2013). *Explain pain* (2nd ed.). Adelaide, Australia: NOI Group Publications.

Clark, M.A., & Lucett, S.C. (2011). *NASM essentials of corrective exercise training*. Philadelphia, PA: Lippincott Williams & Wilkins.

Skarabot, J., Beardsley, C., & Stirn, I. (2015). Comparing the effects of self-myofascial release with static stretching on ankle range-of-motion in adolescent athletes. *International Journal of Sports Physical Therapy, 10*(2), 203-212.

Chapter 3

American Congress of Obstetricians and Gynecologists (ACOG). (2016, May). Frequently asked questions: Exercise during pregnancy. Retrieved from www.acog.org/patients/FAQs/exercise-during-pregnancy.

Stull, K., & Elliott. B. (2015). *Foam rolling: Principles and practices* [Course manual]. TriggerPoint Performance Therapy: Austin, TX.

Chapter 4

Curran, P.F., Fiore, R.D., & Crisco, J.J. (2008). A comparison of the pressure exerted on soft tissue by 2 myofascial rollers. *Journal of Sport Rehabilitation, 17*, 432-442.

Chapter 5

Bowman, K. (2011). *Every woman's guide to foot pain relief: The new science of healthy feet*. Dallas, TX: BenBella Books.

Cooke, M.W., Lamb, S.E., Marsh, J., & Dale, J. (2003). A survey of current consultant practice of treatment of severe ankle sprains in emergency departments in the United Kingdom. *Emergency Medical Journal, 20*(6), 505-507.

Grieve, R., Goodwin, F., Alfaki, M., Bourton, A.J., Jeffries, C., & Scott, H. (2015). The immediate effect of bilateral self myofascial release on the plantar surface of the feet on hamstring and lumbar spine flexibility: A pilot randomized controlled trial. *Journal of Bodywork & Movement Therapies, 19*, 544-552.

Martin, R.L., Davenport, T.E., Reischl, S.F., McPoil, T.G., Matheson, J.W., Wukich, D.K., & McDonough, C.M. (2014). Heel pain—plantar fasciitis: Revision. *Journal of Orthopaedic & Sports Physical Therapy, 44*(11), A1-33.

Neumann, D. (2010). *Kinesiology of the musculoskeletal system: Foundations for rehabilitation*. (2nd ed.). St. Louis, MO: Mosby Elsevier.

Chapter 7

Schleip, R., Duerselen, L., Vleeming, A., Naylor, I.L., Lehmann, H., Zorn, A. . . . Klingler, W. (2012) Strain hardening of fascia: Stat stretching of dense fibrous connective tissue can induce a temporary stiffness increase accompanied by enhanced matrix hydration. *Journal of Bodywork and Movement Therapies, 16*, 94-100.

Thompson, C.R. (2007, January). *Biomechanical approach to the evaluation and treatment of the low back.* Symposium conducted at Eastern Athletic Trainers Association, Boston, MA.

Chapter 8

Clark, M.A., & Lucett, S.C. (2011). *NASM essentials of corrective exercise training.* Philadelphia, PA: Lippincott Williams & Wilkins.

Chapter 9

Silva, L., Andreu, J.L., Munoz, P., Pastrana, M., Millan, I., Sanz, J. . . . Fernandez-Castro, M. (2008). Accuracy of physical examination in subacromial impingement syndrome. *Rheumatology, 47,* 678-683.

Chapter 10

Bell, D.R., Padua, D.A., & Clark, M.A. (2008). Muscle strength and flexibility characteristics of people displaying excessive medial knee displacement. *Archives Physical Medicine and Rehabilitation, 89*(7), 1323-1328.

Cook, G. (2012, October). What is our baseline for movement? Lecture conducted from *the International Federation of Orthopaedic Manipulative Physical Therapists* convention.

Sahrmann, S. (2002). *Diagnosis and treatment of movement impairment syndromes.* St. Louis, MO: Mosby Elsevier.

Chapter 11

ACSM. (2012). Worldwide survey of fitness trends for 2016: 10th anniversary edition. *ACSM's Health & Fitness Journal, 19*(6), 9-18.

Kaneoka, K., Shimizu, K., Hangia, M., Okuwaki, T., Mamizuka, N., Sakaen, M., & Ochiai, N. (2007). Lumbar intervertebral disk degeneration in elite competitive swimmers: A case control study. *American Journal of Sports Medicine, 35*(8), 1341-1345.

Harrison, R.N., Lees, A., McCullagh, P.J., & Rowe, W.B. (1986). A bioengineering analysis of human muscle and joint forces in the lower limbs during running. *Journal of Sports Sciences, 4,* 201-218.

U.S. Department of Labor. (2015). *Nonfatal occupational injuries and illnesses requiring days away from work, 2014.* (USDL Publication No. 15-2205). Washington, DC: U.S. Government Printing Office.

Wolf, B.R., Ebinger, A.E., Lawler, M.P., & Britton, C.L. (2009). Injury patterns in Division I collegiate swimming. *American Journal of Sports Medicine, 10,* 2037-2042.

Chapter 12

McGill, E.A., & Montel, I.N. (Eds.). (2017). *NASM essentials of personal fitness training* (5th ed.). Burlington, MA: Jones & Bartlett.

Chapter 13

Trappe, T.A., White, F., Lambert, C.P., Cesar, D., Hellerstein, M., & Evans, W.J. (2002). Effect of ibuprofen and acetaminophen on postexercise muscle protein synthesis. *American Journal of Physiology, Endocrinology, & Metabolism, 282*(3), E551-E556.

Chapter 14

Grooms, D., Appelbaum, G., & Onate, J. (2015). Neuroplasticity following anterior cruciate ligament injury: A framework for visual-motor training approaches in rehabilitation. *Journal of Orthopaedic & Sports Physical Therapy, 45*(5), 381.

Paterno, M.V., Rauh, M.J., Schmitt, L.C., Ford, K.R., & Hewitt, T.E. (2012). Incidence of contralateral and ipsilateral anterior cruciate ligament (ACL) injury after primary ACL reconstruction and return to sport. *Clinical Journal of Sport Medicine, 22*(12), 116-121.

Rehabilitate. (n.d.). In *Merriam-Webster Online*. Retrieved from www.merriam-webster.com/dictionary/rehabilitate.

Sahrmann, S. (2002). *Diagnosis and treatment of movement impairment syndromes*. St. Louis, MO: Mosby.

ABOUT THE AUTHOR

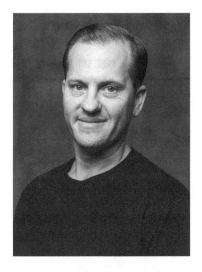

Kyle Stull, DHSc, MS, LMT, CSCS, NASM-CPT, CES, is the senior master trainer and senior manager of research and program design for TriggerPoint, a division of Implus LLC. TriggerPoint is the creator of the GRID Foam Roller and Myofascial Compression Techniques. For the past 13 years, TriggerPoint has helped establish foam rolling as an industry and has advanced the practice forward.

In his position, Kyle collaborates with universities and industry professionals conducting research that provides evidence support for materials that are used for marketing and instructional purposes. Since 2010, he has also been a faculty instructor for the National Academy of Sports Medicine, where he teaches fitness and corrective exercise workshops and contributes content for various journals and articles.

Kyle has achieved a doctorate in health sciences, a master's of science in rehabilitation, and a bachelor's of science in sport management. He is a licensed massage therapist, a certified strength and conditioning specialist, and a corrective exercise specialist with 14 years of experience in personal training, corrective exercise, and manual therapy.

As a member of the Fascia Research Society and the International Academy of Orthopedic Medicine, Kyle is committed to being at the forefront of industry developments and maintaining the highest standards in his practice by incorporating the latest research into his work.

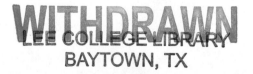

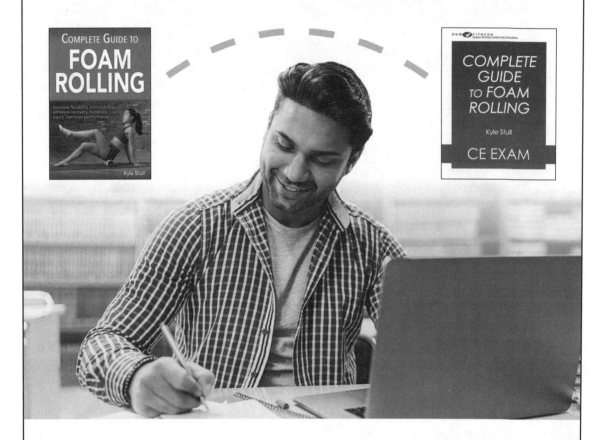
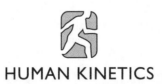